Normal I̶ ̶ ̶ and Bord̶e̶r̶l̶i̶n̶e̶ ̶D̶e̶v̶i̶a̶t̶i̶o̶n̶s̶

Early Diagnosis and Therapy

Inge Flehmig, M. D.

Neuropediatrician
Hamburg, Germany

Foreword by Siegfried M. Pueschel, M. D., Ph. D., M. P. H.

Director, Child Development Center
Brown University Program in Medicine
Providence, Rhode Island, USA

195 illustrations

1992
Georg Thieme Verlag
Stuttgart · New York

Thieme Medical Publishers, Inc.
New York

Inge Flehmig, M.D.
Neuropediatrician
Rothenbaumchaussee 209,
2000 Hamburg 13, Germany

Siegfried M. Pueschel, M.D., Ph.D.,
M. P. H.
Director, Child Development Center
Professor of Pediatrics
Brown University Program in Medicine
Providence, Rhode Island, USA

Photos by Wulf Brackrock, Hamburg

Translated by Roberta Ruben
Schleswiger Str. 2,
2000 Hamburg 50, Germany

Cover design: Dominique Loenicker

*Library of Congress
Cataloging-in-Publication Data*

Flehmig, Inge.
 [Normale Entwicklung des Säuglings und ihre
 Abweichungen. English]
Normal infant development and borderline devia-
tions : early diagnosis and therapy / Inge Flehmig ;
foreword by Siegfried Pueschel.
 p. cm.
Rev. translation of the 4th German ed.: Normale
Entwicklung des Säuglings und ihre Abweichungen.
 Includes bibliographical references and index.
1. Movement disorders in children. 2. In-
fants–Development. 3. Child development devia-
tions. II. Title.
 [DNLM: 1. Cerebral Palsy–diagnosis. 2. Cerebral
Palsy–in infancy & childhood. 3. Cerebral
Palsy–therapy. 4. Child Development. 5. Movement
Disorders–diagnosis. 6. Movement Disorders–in
infancy & childhood. 7. Movement
Disorders–therapy. WS 340 F595n]
RJ496.M68F5413 1992
618.92'83–dc20
DNLM/DLC   92-3158
for Library of Congress   CIP

1st German edition 1979
1st Dutch edition 1982
2nd German edition 1983
1st Bulgarian edition 1987
3rd German edition 1987
1st Latvian edition 1987
1st Portuguese edition 1987
1st Spanish edition 1988
4th German edition 1990

This book is an authorized and revised translation
of the 4th German edition published and copy-
righted 1990 by Georg Thieme Verlag, Stuttgart,
Germany. Title of the German edition: Normale
Entwicklung des Säuglings und ihre Abweichungen, Früherkennung und Frühbehandlung.
Some of the product names, patents and registered
designs referred to in this book are in fact registered trademarks or proprietary names even
though specific reference to this fact is not always
made in the text. Therefore, the appearance of a
name without designation as proprietary is not to
be construed as a representation by the publisher
that it is in the public domain.

© 1992 Georg Thieme Verlag, Rüdigerstraße 14, 7000 Stuttgart 30, Germany
Thieme Medical Publishers, Inc., 381 Park Avenue South, New York, N Y 10016

Typesetting by Setzerei Lihs, D-7140 Ludwigsburg (System 4 mit Linotronic 300)
Printed in Germany by Druckhaus Götz GmbH, D-7140 Ludwigsburg

ISBN 3-13-777301-6 (GTV, Stuttgart)
ISBN 0-86577-428-5 (TMP, New York)   1 2 3 4 5 6

Foreword

A wealth of information is provided in this most valuable volume in a very lucid and succinct way, which will be of great assistance to pediatricians, neurologists, physical therapists, developmental specialists, and other professionals working in child development. This book also incorporates new aspects and recent studies concerning neurodevelopmental issues and thus is a "state-of-the-art" contribution to the field of infant development.

The author describes initially normal motor developmental processes and beautifully illustrates the numerous infantile reactions and their variability. In addition, assessment techniques are masterfully detailed and a classification of neurodevelopmental disabilities is provided. Most importantly, normal developmental processes as they evolve during the first 18 months of life and their deviations are skillfully discussed.

Dr. Flehmig has the talent to translate the present knowledge of early infant development into practical applications and expertly explains in simple terms appropriate as well as inappropriate handling of infants at various ages in different circumstances.

Moreover, this book not only emphasizes early diagnosis and early treatment of affected infants, but also focuses on accurate assessment and proper identification of babies with developmental disabilities. This in turn will often result in improvement of the quality of life of children with neurodevelopmental handicapping conditions.

For her significant contribution to the literature of infant development, Dr. Flehmig ought to be congratulated.

Spring 1992   *Siegfried M. Pueschel, M.D., Ph.D., M.P.H.*

Preface

In the past several years, much has changed in the area of developmental neurology. More in-depth research has not only expanded our knowledge of this subject matter, but is now lending practical aid to pediatricians and general practitioners.

This book is intended as practical help for physicians and therapists in order to make it possible for them to care for the child together and ease it through the early childhood stage.

However, the book is not a scientific paper, but rather a kind of "cookbook" for my fellow pediatricians. It deals with the many-faceted problems which can inevitably arise in cases of infant cerebral damage.

I was not concerned with offering a diagnosis in each case; I wanted to make the reader aware of minute deviations from the breadth of variations of the norm in order to introduce intervention as early as possible. This way, it is not the type of intervention as much as its adaptation to the deviations that is key.

If one waits until all possible diagnoses have been secured, it is often too late to initiate effective therapy. Modern-day therapists are familiar with these interrelations and should make use of the existing options without delay.

Perfectionism was not on my mind while writing this book. I was more concerned with uncovering those tendencies which make the integration of handicapped children into their environment possible or even improve it. Furthermore, I wanted to demonstrate that vantage points for therapy can be found if development and the organism, including its functions, are viewed as a whole. With this book I would like to encourage such a concept. Panta rhei!

I am deeply grateful to the therapists of all areas of expertise, with whom I have enjoyed great cooperation, for the many ideas and knowledge they have shared with me. All our therapeutic knowledge will constantly be challenged through this continuous exchange of experience and persistent testing of how the child in need of treatment can be better helped in mastering its daily problems.

Close contact between child, family, physician, and therapist facilitate reaching a diagnosis. It also makes it possible for the therapist to treat the child more effectively and helps the parents to better handle the often difficult problems they face.

I thank my publisher, Georg Thieme Verlag, for its patience in waiting for the completion of the manuscripts and for the lovely presentation of the book. I thank Roberta Ruben for her smooth and competent translation. Leo Stern holds my deep gratitude for his expert editing of the English manuscript. He completed this task shortly before his death, which came as a shock to all of us and much before its time. My husband and my colleagues earn a very special mention, for without them and their constant support I could not carry out my work.

Spring 1992   *Inge Flehmig, M.D.*

Contents

Introduction

Drawing the borderline between variations of normal infant development and minimal or real deviations from this norm—especially in early infancy—often presents the examiner with considerable diagnostic problems. This book is an attempt to recognize and evaluate early deviations from normal development with the help of illustrations of the continuous progression of infant development in monthly intervals beginning at birth and continuing until the 18th month. Indicating "milestones" of development, as has been done in many cases in the past, is not sufficient for the purpose of this book. Due to the possibilities for treatment of handicapped children, which have been constantly improving in the last few years, the theory is no longer acceptable whereby initially slight abnormalities in an infant's development are just followed to see whether or not they will eventually turn into undeniable handicaps.

The medical examinations for children which were first required by law in 1971 in the Federal Republic of Germany may prove to be advantageous. Nevertheless, if these examinations are to become important with regard to actual early treatment, quite detailed knowledge is needed by the examining pediatricians in clinics and practices. In particular, the initial stages of development during the first months of an infant's life frequently cause problems even for an experienced examiner faced with deciding whether or not a slight abnormality can be dismissed as an insignificant deviation from the norm or should be treated. If the same child is examined by several different physicians, it is not unusual for each one to hold a different opinion with regard to the diagnostic and therapeutic value of the said slight abnormality. This fact can lead to an undesired—and for the child very often disadvantageous—distrust of the parents toward decisions made by physicians.

In order to avoid this and to achieve as uniform a nomenclature and case evaluation as possible, it appears very important to place special emphasis on the examination of the "borderline cases," e.g., between "still normal" and "slightly conspicuous."

Just about every layperson is familiar with the picture of a handicapped individual. However, only with the help of a reliable interpretation of minimal abnormalities will it be possible to recognize minor or—through compensation mechanisms—"concealed" cases of infant handicaps early enough to carry out treatment which can correctly call itself "early." This requires the examining physician to have a certain degree of all-around knowledge of the terminology and possible interpretations of the disorder.

In order to provide the reader of this book—who examines children of various ages—with the opportunity to compare his or her patient's characteristics with normal development for a specified age, the entire spectrum of examinations and observations is illustrated for each month of age. The risk of unavoidable repetition is accepted. If this book is read through continuously (although these chapters were written in chart form and not necessarily intended for continuous reading), the information readily remains in mind due to its repetition.

Due to the fact that after the fourth month of age deviating as opposed to normal development shows a typical uniformity, it was decided to provide comparisons after that point at intervals, namely at 8 and 15 months of age. Retardation may manifest itself during the interim months. For this reason it was decided to forgo continuous repetition of symptomatology, as it would have done more harm than good with regard to understanding of the material.

Early diagnosis of cerebral motor disturbances and other infant disabilities has been increasingly brought forward and extends into the first few months of an infant's life. This has arisen from recognition of the fact that the infant brain is more able to adapt to outside manipulation due to its high level of plasticity than later on. During this period, development of the infant brain follows an almost predictable ability to learn, depending upon its speed of maturation and the stimulation it receives from its environment. Physiotherapeutic measures, therefore, become effective in a more complex and integral manner in this early phase than at a more advanced stage of differentiation of various brain sections, at which time they would only be effective with greater effort.

This book deals with the early diagnosis of infant disabilities resulting from diffuse cerebral damage. Emphasis is placed upon "recognition" and not "diagnosis." Establishing a diagnosis—in the real sense of the term—is not yet possible for a newborn at the beginning of its psychomotor development. Classification of a possible physical handicap or certain diagnosis of a cerebral motor disturbance with regard to its intensity and prognosis appears to be practically impossible at this stage. As a result of years of practice in this special area of child neurology and the observations and discoveries many experienced examiners have made, it is important to point out that, at this early infant age, only "tendencies" can be noted or suspected. These tendencies should catch the examiner's attention and cause him or her to call for evaluations at regular, short intervals or even to introduce suitable therapeutic strategies.

Repeatedly, the thought has been voiced that through this type of early diagnosis many "healthy" children are put through unnecessary early treatment, thus removing therapy places—which are few in number—from those who really need them. Unfortunately, the opposite seems to be true. Despite their detailed experience in this area, all examiners with whom I am acquainted stated that the children under their surveillance became physically and/or behaviorally handicapped and/or developed a learning disability.

The human brain—especially of the infant—seems to possess self-regulating mechanisms which, to a certain degree, are able to compensate for deviations from normal development. These mechanisms are dependent upon the child's immediate environment, that is, upon the extent to which it allows self-regulation or more or less hampers it. Various regulation processes are possible:

- The child regulates itself by including its environment (smiles and cries of demanding character).

- The environment (in most cases the mother) can give counter-regulatory help (in most cases intuitively).

- A physician or therapist may help the mother by showing her methods of "handling" which, in turn, make child–mother self-regulation possible.

- Therapy, along with corresponding treatment techniques, make adaptation through stimulation possible in cases of minor brain damage.

These abnormalities may resurface at certain stages of the child's further development. The beginning of school and the extra pressure this involves for a child up to age 10 years may be one of these critical periods in which abnormal motor development becomes manifest. At this point, perhaps the relatively large number of children with neurogenic learning disabilities should also be mentioned (Stutte 1960, Johnson & Myklebust 1971). Because of this, it seems justified to direct the examiner's attention to tendencies of deviating development and, upon the slightest proof of suspicion, to encourage therapy to be started.

This book's intention is to give pediatricians advice and criteria for the early diagnosis of deviations from normal motor development in order to enable optimum care of the infant presented to them.

A Short Historical Retrospective

On 20 February 1838 Little (1862) performed the first tenotomy described in the literature. He himself suffered from conditions resulting from poliomyelitis which had paralysed his left leg. He was motivated to pursue his goal (the study of medicine) by his own disability, because he believed he could then treat and cure himself. He devoted himself to the study of the "clubfoot" and went to Berlin and other German centers of expertise to study. It soon became clear to him that he suffered from a neuromuscular incoordination, leading to his interest in the surgical treatment of this illness. A surgeon by the name of Stromeyer performed a successful subcutaneous tenotomy of the Achilles tendon on him, after which Little felt healed. Consequently, at the age of 27 and after carrying out many successful operations, he became a "clubfoot" specialist.

In connection with this, he occupied himself intensively with the study of spastic diplegia, which from then on was called "Little's disease." His first publications appeared in *Lancet* in 1844 and 1861. They dealt with the spastic rigidity of the extremities in newborns.

The first description of muscular dystrophy was also written by him. The major contribution was his 1862 monograph entitled "On the Influence of Abnormal Parturition, Difficult Labours, Premature Birth, and Asphyxia Neonatorum on the Mental and Physical Condition of the Child, Especially in Relation to Deformities." He believed that these symptoms of infant cerebral motor disturbance could be diagnosed at the age of 6 months to 2 years. Since he was unable to find any other written work on this subject, he went back to Shakespeare, who in Richard III writes:

I that am curtailed of this fair proportion
Cheated of feature by dissembling Nature,
Deform'd, unfinished, sent before my time
Into this breathing world, scarce half made up,
And that so lamely and unfashionable
That dogs bark at me as I halt by them.
(I,1,18–23)

If ever he have child, abortive be it;
Prodigious and untimely brought to light.
Whose ugly and unnatural aspect
May fright the hopeful mother at the view;
And that be heir to his unhappiness.
(I,2,21–25)

Little was convinced that Shakespeare was describing a person who had suffered asphyxia during birth, apparently in combination with footling presentation and a premature birth.

Freud (1901) describes "Infantile Cerebral Palsy" in several monographs (containing no less than 415 bibliographical references). Treatment was purely medicamentous or surgical. Therapeutic attempts were unsuccessful and without substantial hope for real improvement, expecially in the presence of cerebral seizures. Freud was acquainted with Little's work.

Thereafter, cerebral motor disturbance became an illness which preoccupied mainly orthopedic surgeons—with the exception of neurologists for diagnosis—with the aim of improving the surgical method practiced by Little. Only after the fundamental work of the Bobaths (1952–1975) did it become apparent to the pediatrician that this illness can be therapeutically treated in early childhood.

Fundamental research on the problem of early diagnosis and treatment of cerebral palsy was carried out between 1927 and 1972 by Peiper (1964), Gesell (1941), McGraw (1943), Illingworth (1966), André-Thomas (1952) in cooperation with Sainte-Anne Dargassies (1972) and others. Collis (1964) and particularly Köng (1965) had both dealt mainly with poliomyelitis in their studies during the early 1950s and systematically began to deepen our knowledge regarding cerebral palsy, making early diagnosis possible, which in turn made early therapeutic approaches attainable.

The exact and statistically well-founded research by Prechtl and Beintema (1964) on neurological examinations of newborns up to 15 days of age provided the foundation for systematic examination steps which can easily be followed by every experienced examiner.

In 1974 Bobath stated that he could not recall having heard anything about the clinical picture of "cerebral palsy" during his medical studies. It was not until his wife's physiotherapeutic work confronted him with these problems that he became aware of the disturbances with which one must deal in this illness. The attempt to clarify their connection in what was becoming a visible clinical picture of this illness and the possibilities of therapeutic influence on it determined his further medical activities. This socioeconomically significant syndrome was also either not at all or only partially mentioned during my own medical school studies. Currently, almost all universities offer students opportunities to become acquainted with cerebral motor disturbances in connection with perinatal and neonatal injuries.

Not to be forgotten are Piaget's (1975) basic studies in which he grants *sensomotoricity* the decisive role in the child's development of more complex processes without entirely explaining it.

Jean Ayres (1979) and others, partially building upon their own knowledge, must be given the credit for explaining the expression *sensomotoricity,* which has offered new points of departure for improved therapies.

Normal and Deviating Motor Development

General Notes

The static and motor development of newborns into adults depends on the maturation process of the central nervous system. The process of this development is determined by genetically established patterns of behavior and stimulation from the environment. These stimuli are received by the sensory organs and responded to by the brain, which is an organ of integration and coordination, with automatically flowing complex reactions. These reactions vary, depending on the child's age; however, they do proceed in a fixed sequence beginning at birth. They are characterized by the appearance of the reflex mechanisms of posture and its retention which enable human beings to stand upright and, despite gravity, to keep their balance.

Motor ability provides humans with the possibility of critical interaction with their environment. For the child, the constant improvement in motor functions means achievement of its independence and the ability to adapt to social conditions. The course of motor development interacts directly with psychological and cognitive processes. These processes almost always express themselves through motor behavior, e.g., through facial expression or posture, which has a signal effect upon the environment during the utilization of regulatory processes.

Taking up posture and/or movement and retaining it involve sensorimotor functioning processes in the sense of biological regulatory processes. Perception and movement depend mutually upon each other and should be viewed as a biological unit.

Any sequence of movements is always carried out with optimum adaption to external stimuli. The organism and its environment are dependent upon each other within this regulatory process. According to Schilling (1970), motor ability or the state of motor development always depends upon the environment, meaning it is dependent upon the particular situation.

For Christian (1952) movement is not the result of organs which have become secure in their functioning but rather the utilization of functioning organs.

After birth, all the biological systems endeavor to adapt themselves to the environment. Vital systems such as heartbeat, breathing, etc. achieve this within very a short time, as it is necessary for them to function immediately.

Due to the fact that the human being is born "relatively" too early— since it would be unable to pass through the birth canal if further intrauterine maturation were to take place—less vital systems such as motoricity, statics, etc. require a longer time for postpartum adaption. Preparation takes place during pregnancy and birth.

Here we are not dealing with simple systems which spontaneously change from their original immaturity to their final maturity but rather with patterns which are constantly subject to self-regulation. These adapt themselves to the situation at any given time, and thus they learn to operate with the means at their disposal with regard to a given pattern which has become genetically memorized.

What means does, for example, motor activity use? Here, regulation of tone seems to be in the foreground: inhibition of lower brain centers and stimulation of more highly integrated centers through finely graded regulation and counter-regulation which always influence each other. No stage can be attained without first having passed through the preceding one. In this manner, a genetically memorized pattern along with the environmental stimuli, which partially hamper and partially channel this development, comes to full blossom.

The fact that this complicated system can show defects in its operation through a multitude of very different disorders is due to its numerous regulating systems. Its coordinated interaction within the microcosm of a developing child with its psyche, with its ability to react to stimuli from its environment, with the possibilities opened by its sensory sensitive systems and its intellect of not always reacting to those stimuli in a preconceived way, all this means having a certain amount of freedom of reaction which leads to what we call "development."

Only a very small portion is visible to the examiner and only becomes comprehensible when one system no longer functions, for example, as a result of brain damage. Due to the regulatory failure, the organism is faced with a new situation which it can only master by modifying some mechanisms of adaption. Since these are no longer completely genetically preprogrammed, the system must find a way to make adaption as optimal as possible.

A damaged system that has not yet fully matured will have a better chance for adaptation than a system which is already completely mature and has "fixed" channels that are no longer open. This is what is called the brain's "plasticity" or "dynamism," which is most fertile during the first months of life. The further an organism is developed, the more numerous are its reactions, and the easier it is to disturb the entire system. This system is developed in such a way that in transition from one type of reaction to another—suitably adjusted to changing conditions—previous experience is programmed to leave its mark.

Reactions of Motor Behavior

According to Peiper (1964), the receptors of postural sense and kinesthesia serve the development of static and motor capabilities. The position of the limbs in comparison with each other and—with the body in an upright position—the position of the head, body, and limbs with regard to the direction of gravity is subject to constant surveillance and correction. In this case the receptors are the pressure sense organs of the skin, the proprioceptors of muscles, tendons, and joints, the eyes, and the internal ear with its system of balance and hearing. In order to fulfill the same task, various sense organs become active simultaneously. Thus, numerous reactions are covered several times over.

During the course of an infant's statomotor development, certain regular patterns become apparent which are linked to the development of the fetal brain. The various parts of the brain begin to function in the same sequence in which these develop.

From the information gathered by analysis of the reflexes and reactions appearing during the first year of life, the brain's blueprint can be delineated (McGraw 1943). The characteristics of behavior of newborns show that they are under the dominance of subcortical nuclei. These mature at an earlier stage than the cortex of the brain. The behavior of the newborn and infant is, therefore, characterized by these primary patterns. Some of these patterns remain under their influence at a later age. Following further maturation of the brain, these primary behavioral patterns become hindered. The process of development takes place in a craniocaudal direction. It can best be demonstrated through the appearance and disappearance of reactions in interaction with normal motor development as shown in Table **1** and Figures **1–16**.

Table 1   Reactions and motor behavior

Reaction	Days			Months													
	1	2	3	1	2	3	4	5	6	7	8	9	10	11	12	13	14
Magnet reaction																	
Stepping reaction																	
Placing reaction																	
Galant reaction																	
Glabella reaction																	
Doll's-eyes phenomenon																	
Neck positioning reaction																	
Moro reaction (1st and 2nd phase)																	
Bauer's reaction																	
TLR (tonic labyrinthine reaction) (in prone position)																	
ATNR (asymmetric tonic neck reaction)																	
Palmar grasp reaction																	
Plantar grasp reaction																	
LR (labyrinthine placing reaction)																	
Lateral position reaction																	
Landau's reaction																	
Placing reaction — Head respective to body and body respective to body; Initial raising into upright position for sitting; Turning, beginning rotation																	
Raising of head from supine position																	
Readiness reaction (parachute reaction)																	
Balance reaction: Prone position																	
Supine position																	
With front support in sitting position																	
With lateral support in sitting position																	
With back support in sitting position																	
Balance on all fours (crawling)																	
Standing without balance																	
Standing with balance																	
Walking without balance																	
Walking with balance																	

This table is a nonstandardized survey

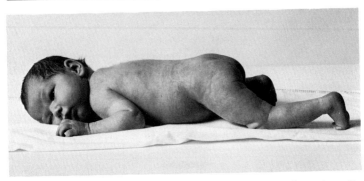

Fig. **1 Automatic reaction.** A newborn in a prone position always turns its head to one side—usually onto the same side—in order to keep its respiratory tract patent. Here, we are dealing with a first extension from total flexion

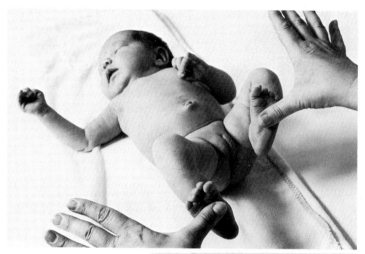

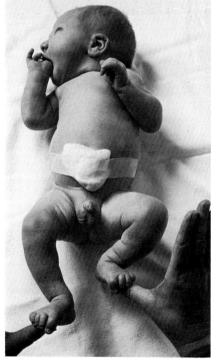

Fig. **2 a, b Magnet reaction.**
In a supine position with bent
hips and knees (symmetrical
position of head in the center
line), the examiner presses
his or her thumbs onto the
soles of the infant's feet and
slowly pulls the thumbs
back. Contact is kept be-
tween soles and fingers. The
legs stretch; the feet seem to
be "glued" to the fingers

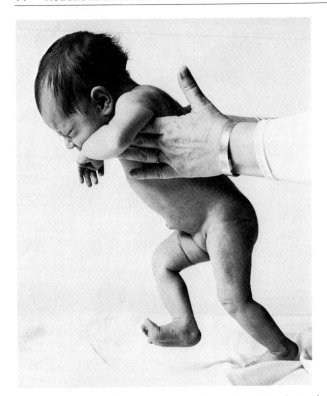

Fig. **3** **Stepping reaction.** The child is held up vertically by the trunk with both hands. If the sole of one foot is pressed onto the underlying surface, the corresponding leg will bend upon contact and the other will stretch. The stretched foot then touches the surface, the leg bends, and the previously bent leg then stretches. This alternating movement gives the impression of stepping (marche automatique). The upper part of the child's body is tilted slightly forward

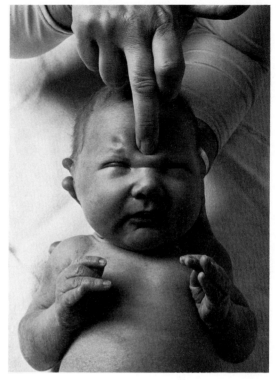

Fig. **4   Glabella reaction.** If pressure is applied to the middle of the forehead, the eyes close. According to Prechtl and Beintema, pareses of the facial nerve becomes visible this way

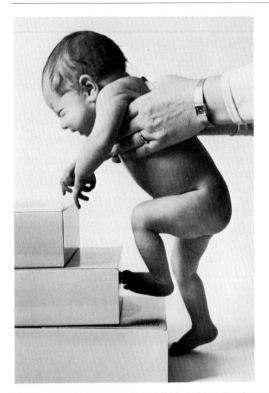

Fig. **5   Placing reaction.** The child is held under the arms with its feet under the edge of a table. The child is slowly lifted in such a way that the instep of its foot slightly touches the bottom edge of the table, and, as a result, the foot "climbs" over the table's edge. This reaction can also be triggered with the back of the hand. This reaction is also called the climbing reaction, since the child gives the impression of being able to climb over the edge of the table

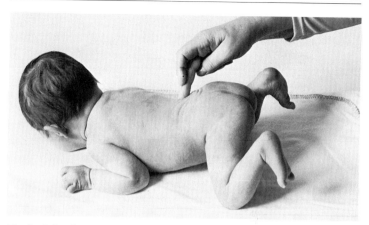

Fig. 6 **Galant's reaction.** If the child is stroked paravertebrally with one finger, its body curves. The concavity proceeds toward the direction of the stimulus; the pelvis is raised. The corresponding leg and arm are stretched, the opposite extremities are curved. This reaction is often also called the spinal reaction

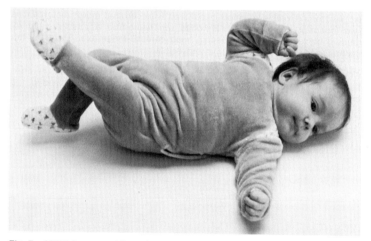

Fig. 7 **ATNR (asymmetric tonic neck reaction).** If the child's head is turned to one side, the extremities of the "facial side" are stretched, and the extremities of the "occipital side" are bent. This is the so-called "fencer's position." In most cases this reaction produces only one effect on the extremities, which can be demonstrated electromyographically. If it persists, hand-eye coordination is hampered. It is found in children with cerebral disturbance of movement. Due to its tonically fixed posture, it renders all movement against gravity impossible

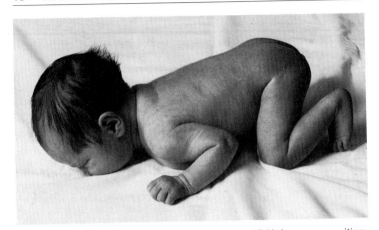

Fig. 8   **TLR (tonic labyrinthine reaction).** When the child is in a prone position, there is a total curve. The head is not turned to one side, the respiratory tract is not kept patent. In the supine position, the child's trunk and legs are stretched. The strech is adducted and internally rotated. The arms are bent, the hands close into fists, the shoulders are retracted. The head is in an opisthotonic position. To a very minor extent this is present in normal infants. This is the most common visible reaction in children with cerebral motor disturbances (e.g., quadriplegia). It prevents the child from rising from a dorsal position by holding back the head and making head control impossible. Since the hip cannot be bent, balanced sitting is impossible

STNR (symmetric tonic neck reaction). If the child's head is bent, the arms bend at the elbows, and the legs are stretched. If the head is extended, the arms are stretched, and the legs are bent. Should this reflex persist, it hampers the tetrapod stand and with it the ability to sit up

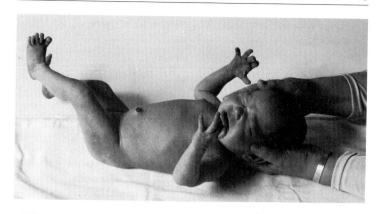

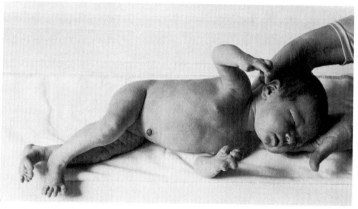

Fig. **9a, b Neck righting reaction.** The examiner turns the lying child's head to one side. The child's entire body follows the turn; the child turns en bloc. Should this reaction persist, rotation between head and body and, with this, sitting up from a supine position with the help of turning, becomes impossible

Lateral position reaction. The child is held vertically at the trunk with both hands around the waist and moved sideways into a horizontal position. The head again adjusts itself within the space; the upper leg and arm are stretched, whereas the lower extremities are bent. Through passive sinking of the head, the child's entire body collapses. This pattern can also be observed in reactions of balance in the adult

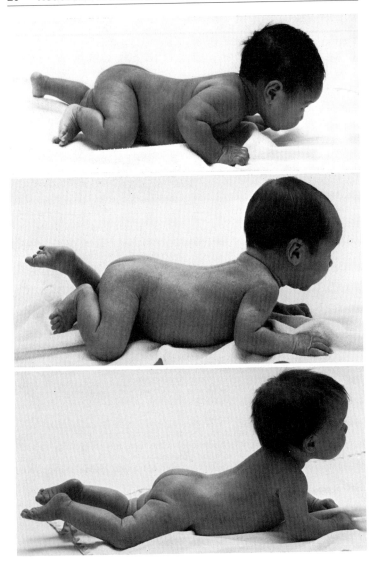

Fig. 10a–c Labyrinthine righting reaction. When the child is laid on its abdomen or its position is changed within a given space, the child's head adjusts itself to the surroundings; the child raises its head. This reaction can also be triggered in a head-down position. In some children with cerebral disturbances of movement this is missing and results in lack of head control

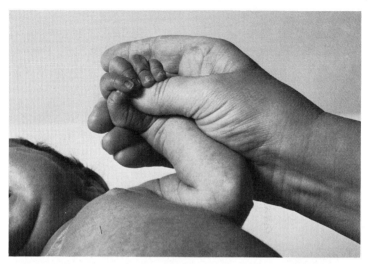

Fig. **11** **Palmar grasp reaction.** Contact with the palm of the hand stimulates the hand to close. As long as this stimulus remains, the hand may remain closed. It is possible to pull the child upward by the hands in this position. The elbow joints remain slightly bent. Should this reaction persist for a substantial amount of time, the child will not be able to support itself on its open palms (no balance reactions). This becomes physiologically strengthened through sucking

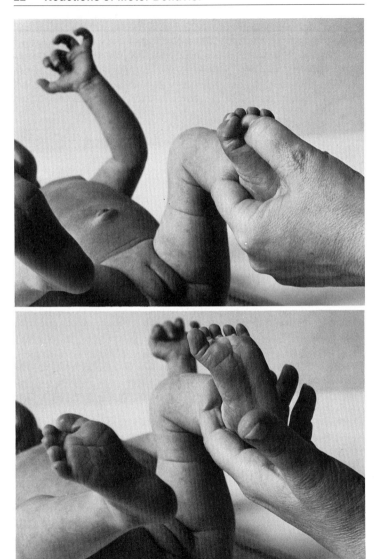

Fig. **12a, b Plantar grasp reaction.** Contact with the balls of the feet causes the toes to clutch together. When the contact is removed, the toes spread apart. Should this reaction persist, standing on flat feet and walking (including the rolling movement) are not possible

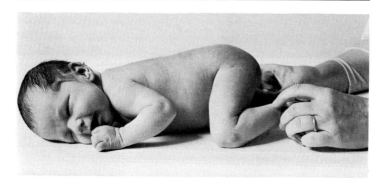

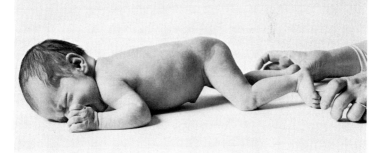

Fig. **13a, b   Bauer reaction.** If the child is lying in prone position and the examiner presses his/her thumbs against the soles of the child's feet, the child will begin to crawl, alternating its legs (sometimes even without stimulation)

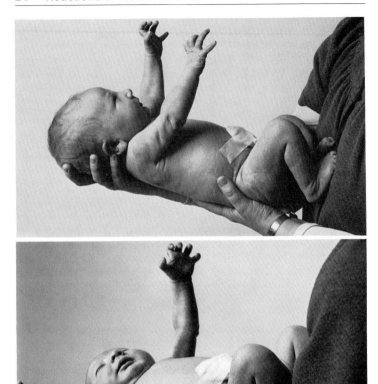

Fig. **14a, b   Moro reaction.** For this examination, lay the child upon one fore-
arm and support its head with the other hand. Then the hand holding the child's
head is lowered. The child's head falls into the opened hand. The child opens its
mouth, the arms are lifted and opened, the fingers are stretched apart like a fan
(1st phase). Then the mouth is closed again, the arms are bent and joined
together again in front of the child's body (2nd phase). Should this condition
persist, the child will not be able to learn to sit or to close its mouth in order to eat
or speak. Saliva is not swallowed, so the child slobbers. While the child's head is
in the mid-line at the starting point of this test, an asymmetry may be an
indication of a paresis on one side. One must be certain that the child is not lying
in the ATNR position. It is important here to wait before triggering this reaction.
The Moro reaction is always seen spontaneously when the child suddenly loses
its balance. This can also be observed occasionally in adults

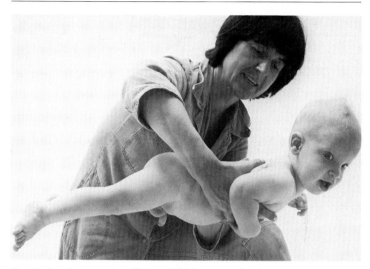

Fig. **15 Landau reaction.** If the child is suspended horizontally—with the examiner's hands wrapped round its trunk—the child will automatically lift its head and the legs follow this movement by extending (craniocaudal). Should the head suddenly bend, the child's entire body bends. This reaction is necessary for a few months during the first year of life in order for the child to experience the feeling of its body in a given area (bodyschema)

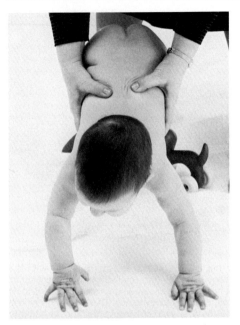

Fig. **16** **Parachute reaction.** The examiner holds the infant with both hands around the waist at the trunk and lowers its head relatively fast to the surface below. Before the head reaches the surface the arms are extended (optical readiness to jump), and later the transfer of body weight to the arms occurs. Just as the readiness to stand belongs to the reactions of balance, so does this the parachute reaction and remains for life. Typical fractures of the radius are the result of this reaction

Sucking and swallowing reactions. According to Peiper, the newborn begins to suck at the very first food intake, and immediately thereafter it begins to swallow. In breastfed infants these reactions tend to persist a bit longer, until they are replaced by voluntary swallowing

Searching reaction. If the child is hungry, it moves its head without external stimuli. If a corner of the child's mouth is touched by a finger or any other item (e.g., a bottle), the child's head turns in the direction of the stimulus (rooting reaction, réflexe des points cardinaux)

Doll's-eyes phenomenon. If the child's head is slowly turned, the eyes move in the opposite direction; if the movement is fast, a nystagmus may be triggered. According to Illingworth, abducens paresis becomes visible through asymmetry of this response

Summary: Interpretation of Reactions

The essential developmental factor of infant motor behavior is the emergence of the *reflex mechanism for the reactions of posture*. For this the following are required:

- Reactions of righting and balance
- Modification of primary, primitive, synergic mass movements into specialized, individual movements
- Development of a gradually changing muscle tone for withstanding gravity

The *posture reflex mechanisms* bring about head control within space, positioning of the head with regard to the trunk, and positioning of the trunk with regard to the extremities through rotation and/or adaptation of agonists and antagonists. The human being's capabilities to hold itself in an upright position, manipulate itself agilely, speak and think call for a mechanism for maintaining posture and for coordinating the respective patterns of movement. This occurs automatically and is adapted to the requirements of the moment.

The development of these mechanisms requires a certain amount of *time for adaptation*. This adaptation is made possible through the following factors:

- Normal posture tone
- Normal reciprocal innervation for
  a) A more intricate gradation of movement
  b) Adjusted contraction between the flexors and extensors in order to achieve the necessary fixation which is the prerequisite for precision in movement
  c) Normal patterns of coordination

A normal reflex mechanism for maintaining posture is the guarantee for normal movement which is common to all human beings.

The following belong to the group referred to as placing reactions:

- Labyrinthine righting reaction onto the head
- Neck righting reaction
- Body righting reaction respective to head
- Body righting reaction respective to body
- Optical righting reaction

The *reactions of balance* deal with automatic, unconscious fluctuations of visible countermovements. The body's muscles are continuously adjusted in order to maintain balance, which means securing the quality of motor ability achieved through the righting reaction. Modification of the primary, primitive, synergistic mass movements to specialized, individual movements is achieved through dissociation and/or emancipation of the individual joints which, as a result, achieve the ability to operate separately, permitting more intricate manipulation. The developing individual learns to inhibit all of its patterns of movement in order to modify them for more intricate ones. This is only made possible through the constantly changing and adapting muscle tone—the factor which allows the infant to raise itself despite the force of gravity. Certain joints, such as the hip, attain an important position as they must react dissociatedly as well as under the pressure of weight.

Muscle tone regulation is not exclusively assured by the interaction of receptors and their regulatory systems within the muscles, tendons, and joints or through sensation by way of the skin regarding positioning in space. It is, above all, secured through the vestibular system with its connections to the eyes and ears.

No sensorimotor system of perception seems to possess such a high value as does the above-mentioned vestibular system, as it is fundamental for the upright position in space; i.e., it is responsible for being "human" as such. No sensorimotor system of perception is so preprogramed, learned, and/or practiced as this regulatory system. Breakdowns within the vestibular system with its nuclei and pathways and connections to other systems are critically important to recognize, e.g., with regard to the psyche (fright, insecurity, disorientation within space and time).

Ascertainable Motor Functions during the Examination of Young Infants

A young infant born without the ability to move against gravity and with an almost total lack of head control takes on in all positions a symmetrical bending position which is only occasionally overcome, corresponding to the intrauterine position it held for months. When moving passively, the newborn's head nearly always uncontrollably falls in a ventral, dorsal, or lateral direction. As the brain matures, the child is able to lift its head and stretch its body. Along with improving head control and the extension of the body, the child achieves the ability to perform rotation between the head and the shoulders and between the shoulders and hips. Trunk control improves, and with the increasing support function of the arms and legs, the reactions of balance prepare to unfold to their full function.

These reactions of equilibrium are a further developmental step towards the goal of movement against the force of gravity, to hold balance only with the trunk and legs, leaving the hands free for more intricate manipulation. The ability to differentiate movement develops parallel to the gradual upright movement against the pull of gravity; each of these developments has an influence upon the other.

The ability to execute extension and flexion movements of the extremities develops out of the almost total flexion of the arms and legs through the disappearance of primary reactions, for example, tonic patterns of posture, and irrespective of posture as well as of head movement. As a result, the arms and hands can be used for grasping and the legs and feet, for walking. The continuation of this development process is marked by a sophistication of the sequence of movements. Differentiated movements in an upright position are made possible by the continually improving control of balance. These movements would not develop in such a finely graded manner without a certain self-activating motivation within the child itself to attain an upright position, in addition to the preprogramming of motor development. Through genetically established patterns of behavior—such as the mother–child relationship which has a very high position in this program of development—in its interaction with the environment and the stimulation it contains, the child's desire to achieve an upright position is awakened.

In a *supine position,* the flexion pattern of a child only a few days old is occasionally interrupted if the head changes its isolated position. If the head is passively turned to one side, the trunk follows in the flexion pattern en bloc (neck righting reaction; Fig. **9a–c**). The arms are loosely angled, and the thumbs are sometimes tucked under. Occasionally the hands are open, reinforced by the Moro reaction, which involves extension of the fingers. The trunk can stretch every now and again, the legs extend from the hips outward into an alternating stretch, the child kicks. The arms and legs can be abducted and the feet dorsiflexed and turned out.

In a *prone position*, the newborn frees its respiratory tract by extending and turning the head to the side (automatic reaction; Fig. **1**). Trunk, hip, and knees are bent and the feet dorsiflexed. The head may occasionally be lifted but is still insecure. Due to the slowly developing extension ability the child is better able to bring its arms foreward out of the shoulder and to open its hands. Through the advancing cranio-caudal extension, whole patterns become alternating, symmetrical, independent movements with flexion and extension. This progressing extension mechanism and the increasing control of the position of the head, which can gradually be maintained without outside help, make more extensive movement in the shoulder joints possible.

The child is able to position its head correctly within space. The arms, which are becoming more freely movable, are placed in front so that the forearms can be used for taking on the body weight for support purposes. Simultaneous with the extension in the shoulder area, there is an extension in the trunk and/or hip area. This is the first prerequisite for hip extension, which is necessary for standing later.

All dependent joints become more freely moveable at all levels. Before the end of the first 6 months, the symmetrical posture may be changed. This is required for the introduction to the first turning movements. Grasping with one hand becomes possible when, at approximately the same time, hand-eye coordination develops. In the supine position, the hands are joined at the midline. The child gets to know its body through touching. This bending in the supine position and the stretching of the body in the prone position call into existence the initial ability to move freely against gravity and, with this, to develop both body image and a feeling for correct positioning within space.

The child observes its immediate environment through head and eye movements. The hand soon turns out of the prone position by supination opening the ulnar side, with thumb opposition and advancing of the shoulder. The hands begin to perform more delicate movements and are no longer needed for support purposes.

At the end of a child's first year of life, its body possesses the ability not only to change its posture but also to retain it. The infantile reflexes and reactions retreat more and more. Normal motor development of the infant is dependent upon the continuing process of development already mentioned. Noxious events which lead to a brain lesion may cause disturbances within this sequence of development.

Data on Normal Development with Consideration Given to the Corresponding Age Groups (Denver Developmental Scales)

Although it becomes clear from the preceding that it is very difficult to put a timetable on sequences of development because a multitude of factors influence, for example, the ability to rise from a horizontal into a vertical position, it nevertheless seems useful to indicate certain time-related intervals. Countless attempts have been made to produce charts which list punctual development. This was useful during the years in which early diagnosis was virtually unknown. In the Anglo-American literature the term "milestones" is used for such records in order to characterize in which ways a normal child in various age groups can seemingly predictably move into the upright position.

The one aspect that is not taken into consideration in most charts is the *variation of the norm* and its dependence upon the basic genetic pattern and upon the stimulation and/or motivation by the environment. Charts which have been compiled according to more recent test results do show this variation from the norm, whereby only the point in time of the child's movement out of the horizontal and into the vertical are named, but the *quality of the movements* is not considered (Table **2**).

Greater reliability with regard to the therapeutic possibilities currently offered by neurological developmental treatment lies in the observation of development by means of **motoscopy.** This method makes it possible to examine closely the process of a single movement with special emphasis placed upon its quality; the movement is performed by the child before the examiner's eyes upon his/her request. Here, we are dealing with active participation by the child as opposed to the classically passive neurological examination, for example, of passive resistance or testing of automatic and induced reactions. It is not until we are able to observe the patient perform a series of movements on his/her own that the opportunity arises to analyse the normal processes and the deviations from them.

The concept of the development scales must be altered with regard to early diagnosis. It must be limited to recording only "tendencies of development." Furthermore, it is necessary to become more intensively concerned with the *quality* of a child's attempts to raise itself against the force of gravity.

Table **2**   Denver developmental screening test (STO = stomach, SIT = sitting)

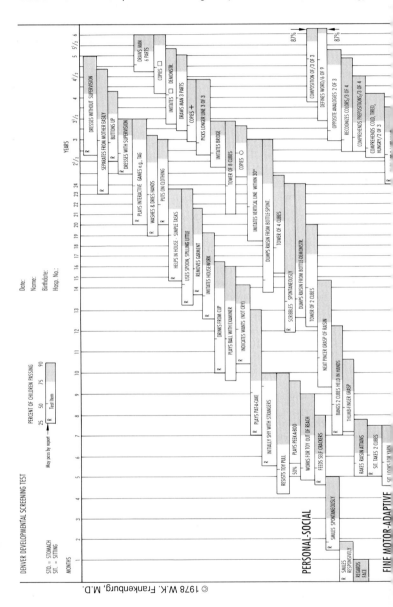

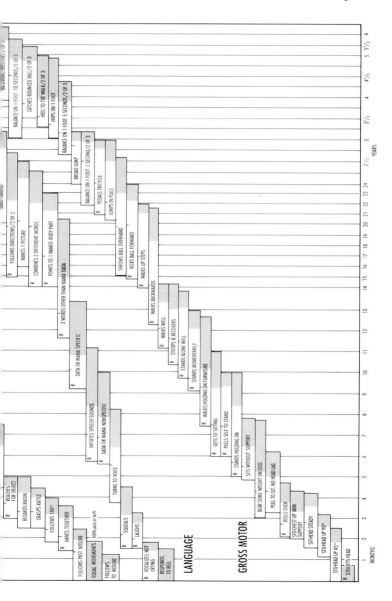

DIRECTIONS

DATE
NAME
BIRTHDATE
HOSP. NO.

1. Try to get child to smile by smiling, talking, or waving to him. Do not touch him.
2. When child is playing with toy, pull it away from him. Pass if he resists.
3. Child does not have to be able to tie shoes or button in the back.
4. Move yarn slowly in an arc from one side to the other, about 6″ (15 cm) above child's face. Pass if eyes follows 90° to midline. (Past midline; 180°)
5. Pass if child grasps rattle when it is touched to the backs or tips of fingers.
6. Pass if child continues to look where yarn disappeared or tries to see where it went. Yarn should be dropped quickly from sight from tester's hand without arm movement.
7. Pass if child picks up raisin with any part of thumb and a finger.
8. Pass if child picks up raisin with the ends of thumb and index finger using an overhand approach.

9. Pass any enclosed form.
   Fail continuous round motions.

10. Which line is longer? (Not bigger.) Turn paper 90° and repeat. (3/3 or 5/6)

11. Pass any crossing lines.

12. Have child copy first. If failed, demonstrate.

When giving items 9, 11, and 12, do not name the forms. Do not demonstrate 9 and 11.

13. When scoring, each pair (2 arms, 2 legs, etc.) counts as one part.
14. Point to picture and have child name it. (No credit is given for sounds only.)
15. Tell child to: Give block to Mommie; put block on table; put block on floor. Pass 2 of 3. (Do not help child by pointing, moving head or eyes.)
16. Ask child: What do you do when you are cold? .. hungry? ..tired? Pass 2 of 3.
17. Tell child to: Put block **on** table; **under** table; **in front** of chair, **behind** chair. Pass 3 of 4. (Do not help child by pointing, moving head or eyes.)
18. Ask child: If fire is hot, ice is _?; Mother is a woman, Dad is a _?; a horse is big, a mouse is _?. Pass 2 of 3.

19. Ask child: What is a ball? .. lake? .. desk? .. house? .. banana? .. curtain? .. ceiling? .. hedge? .. pavement? Pass if defined in terms of use, shape, what it is made of, or general category (such as banana is fruit, not just yellow). Pass 6 of 9.

20. Ask child: What is a spoon made of? .. a shoe made of? .. a door made of? (No other objects may be substituted.) Pass 3 of 3.

21. When placed on stomach, child lifts chest off table with support of forearms and/or hands.

22. When child is on back, grasp his hands and pull him to sitting. Pass if head does not hang back.

23. Child may use wall or rail only, not person. May not crawl.

24. Child must throw ball overhand 3 feet to within arm's reach of tester.

25. Child must perform standing broad jump over width of test sheet. (8–½", 22 cm)

26. Tell child to walk forward,   ∞∞∞∞→   heel within 1" (2,5 cm) of toe.
   Tester may demonstrate. Child must walk 4 consecutive steps, 2 out of 3 trials.

27. Bounce ball to child who should stand 3 feet (1 m) away from tester. Child must catch ball with hands, not arms, 2 out of 3 trials.

28. Tell child to walk backward,   ←∞∞∞∞   toe within 1" (2,5 cm) of heel.
   Tester may demonstrate. Child must walk 4 consecutive steps, 2 out of 3 trials.

DATE AND BEHAVIORAL OBSERVATIONS (how child feels at time of test, relation to tester, attention span, verbal behavior, self-confidence, etc.):

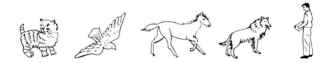

Significance of Sensorimotor Development for the Overall Development of Newborns and Infants

The preceding development scale allows for recognition of the rapid change in motor ability, especially during infancy. Even though this does not enable registration of the state of developmental steps, it does provide an opportunity to locate deviations from the norm.

In this connection, Piaget (1975) speaks of the sensorimotor intelligence a child possesses as a result of heredity. This aspect, in interaction with the child's environment and the progressive use of acquired experience, leads to characteristic behavior. Sensorimotor function makes the power of recognition possible which the child constantly needs in order to adapt to the objects and events in its environment. Piaget calls this process "recognizing and generalizing assimilation."

Furthermore, it seems justified to inquire into the function of the indicated reactions and not only to describe their appearance and/or disappearance, that is not to consider only reflexes or similar items.

What could the significance of reactions of righting and posture be? Which function forms the basis for the reactions of balance? With regard to this, it must be stressed again that during infancy it is hardly possible to separate motor and mental development. Piaget and other authors repeatedly stress the fact that the mental development of a newborn or infant during the first 18 months depends on its ability to move normally. Normal motor development for its part affects the environment and stimulates it to react appropriately. The child's mental and psychological horizon grows out of the interplay of action and reaction. The decisive step toward this broadening of the horizon is seen in the child's raising its body into an upright position.

The righting reactions, which make it possible for a human being to lift its head and stand upright, as well as the mechanisms of posture retention, therefore constitute significant steps for the further development of differentiated motor abilities and also of the mental-psychological development of the human being. Deviations from this can prevent adaptation and make normal development of perception and recognition impossible. It must be clearly emphasized that the inability to recognize one's environment is due to a sensorimotor disturbance. It can be shown in thalidomide children with deformations only of the extremities that they are indeed quite able to develop adequate tactile perception because their senses are not necessarily disturbed. On the other hand, in children with cerebral motor disturbances, there is always a sensorimotor disturbance.

In the reflex arrangement of early infancy, Piaget sees a well-organized and orderly process, which characteristically sustains itself through activity, and as a result sooner or later functions on its own (repetition), assimilates those objects which are suited for this function (generalizing assimilation), and learns to distinguish situations which correspond to certain specific aspects of its activity (motor recognition).

Hence, progressive adaptation of the reflex patterns require their organization and structure. The reflex mechanism can become reinforced through practice or decline as a result of lack of practice, because the laws of reflex activity cause coordination to be connected and effected.

Here we seem to be dealing with a special type of learning process; in a way it resembles an autodidactic process rather than actual acquisition. Piaget writes that those learning processes which are connected to a reflex mechanism pull along behind them a very complex play of forces such as accommodation and assimilation, utilizing individually different structures within the boundaries defined by ourselves. Since the reflex mechanism—without taking note of anything pertaining to the environment as such—still requires this environment, an accommodation process is produced. Even with regard to quite primitive reflex mechanisms, a type of learning seems to take place which, apart from a certain number of hereditary factors, requires an individual consideration of experience.

It becomes obvious that, as mentioned above, a motor matrix must exist and that the development of normal muscle tone, obstruction of tonic patterns of posture and of primary reactions, emergence of righting and balancing reactions, etc. depend to a great extent on the manipulation which the newborn experiences through its mother and/or environment (tactile-kinesthetic-vestibular perception).

Who among us is not familiar with children who suffer from social deprivation and lie quietly and listlessly in their beds without raising themselves from the horizontal to the vertical position on their own? For those of us who have had the opportunity to see how rapidly these children are able to make up for their lack of motor development through intensive stimulation—although the quality of movement is most likely not quite as good as it would be without social deprivation—the great importance environmental stimulation has becomes very clear.

It is true that these are conspicuous deviations, but they look different from cerebral motor disturbances. Nowadays, we know precisely that any deviations from normal motor development in early and even late infancy can lead to a type of motor disability. However, we are also aware that—contrary to the above—good stimulation through the environment produces positive effects on the quality of motor development.

At this point it must be stressed that the main issue at hand is not just the fact that the child moves, but rather in how well coordinated a manner these movements are carried out. Each improvement positively influences the child's ability to process correctly its experience of the environment.

The foundation of movement is sensorimotor perception. Sensorimotor activity must be understood as a regulatory system composed of exteroception and proprioception through the skin (tactile), tendons, muscles, joints, and the vestibular system with its connections to e.g., the visual and auditory systems. In each of these systems, there is external and self-mediation, the differing influences of which must not be overlooked as there is clear relationship to them with regard to therapy and/or stimulation through the environment and the child's reaction to it (behavior, psyche).

Criteria for the Early Diagnosis of Deviating Motor Development in Infancy

In the preceding chapters, normal infant development was described. In the second part of this book, the monthly stages of development are dealt with in more detail. Deviations from this normal development do not necessarily mean that the child must inevitably develop a manifest handicap. However, as we have already mentioned earlier, it is no longer justified—due to our present standard of knowledge—to sit back and wait, i.e., to refrain from becoming actively involved in a specific course of treatment that could alleviate possible pathological development.

In order to do so, it is necessary to establish reliable criteria by which one can single out the discrete findings most likely to develop later into a handicap from the multitude of individual variations of psychomotor development. For simplicity's sake, it should be assumed that in every newborn there is a kind of genetically founded matrix which steers the gradual step-by-step change from the initial horizontal to the vertical position in life—a change which takes place during the first several months of life. Should this matrix be destroyed or damaged through any type of injury, a "severely handicapped" child is the result. In such a case, early diagnosis of the illness is relatively easy and quite obvious to observant, even untrained persons such as the child's parents.

Often the barely distinguishable findings in young infants with "medium" or "minimal" disturbances are recognized too late or not at all by the parents, and frequently not even by specially trained physicians or persons trained in recognizing such nuances in adults or older children. Early diagnosis and correct interpretation of the discrete features of a minimally handicapped child require highly specialized experience which can be gained only by intense work with infants and not through even the most highly specialized literature.

First and foremost, it is more important to gain knowledge about the significance of the degree and ranking order of conspicuous findings in their entirety than it is to identify the individual features themselves. This knowledge alone makes it possible to draw a line between conspicuous findings in need of treatment and the numerous and often conspicuous-looking variations of the wide range of the stages of normal infant development. This knowledge represents the examiner's actual wealth of experience.

The *criteria for early diagnosis* listed in the following merely represent an attempt to give examiners a guideline to work with in order to avoid missing anything during the initial examination of newborns. It is also intended to draw attention to the sometimes hidden deviations of normal development.

The result of the first examination often determines what further steps are to be taken and is, therefore, of major importance. If the examiner finds the child to be suspect in any manner, further short-term examinations should follow. If the child then appears to be healthy, these follow-ups are usually dropped. If the relatively discrete findings in an only slightly affected child are underestimated, a follow-up exam often does not take place until much later when the symptoms have become obvious even to the parents who had been calmed by the initial examination. Instead of optimum early treatment, a child like this might obtain only belated therapy. The disadvantages can be seen in the less effective compensation for damage despite longer and more intensive treatment which, of course, also means higher costs.

With regard to the importance of early examinations, each examiner should compile a sort of checklist which is continuously present during examinations and which can be checked off point-by-point down to the final diagnosis. Experts doubtlessly have their own personal pattern of examining based upon their experience. The importance and ranking order of some individual findings are most likely differently interpreted by different examiners.

The list of criteria for early diagnosis, therefore, does not claim to be universally valid. However, it has proven itself in practical application on thousands of children during the course of a number of years. It is described as being the workable model of a relatively easily executable method of evaluation within the scope of the neurological motor examination.

Criteria for early diagnosis

- Changes in posture and/or muscle tone
- Inadequate or lack of righting reaction
- Inadequate or lack of balancing reaction
- Persistent or tonic patterns of posture which hamper coordination of movement
- Asymmetries in posture which exceed the physiological limits allowed by cerebral dominance
- Developmental delays in all abilities or in partial performances
- Suspected cases of disturbances in the visual, auditory, tactile-kinesthetic areas of perception through lack of sensory integration

● Distracted look and no eye contact despite normal sight

● No sure reaction to noises since localization is not possible, or exaggerated reaction to noise (hyperacousia) despite normal hearing. These children often hold their ears closed when hearing noises of normal loudness.

● Overly sensitive to touch, change in position; behavior tends to be chaotic and psychotic; usually symmetrical hypertonia or adynamia due to lack of sensation in muscles, tendons, and joints is present; low sensitivity to pain; general tone is lax; sometimes frightened if unable to differentiate stimuli originating from the body or from the surroundings; or the child is careless and does not recognize danger as hardly any information reaches it.

Postural and/or muscle tone changes are relatively easy to recognize during the course of the examination. During observation, the child is placed in a dorsal position either more bowed in comparison with the norm—meaning that the head and legs may be raised—or there is more of a stretch—meaning that the child may be in a opisthotonic position. If the child prefers the bowed position, any movement to place him/her into a new position can only be undertaken en bloc. In the stretched position, all attempts at rotation are difficult. The shoulders are extensively retracted, the arms are in a prone position, the hands are balled into fists with turned in and adducted thumbs. If the child prefers the bowed position, it may be difficult or impossible for the child to raise itself or to turn its head sideways when in an abdominal position.

In newborns, the only **righting reaction** possible is the neck righting reaction. After approximately 3 months it disappears and is replaced by the righting reactions of the head towards the body and by the reactions of the body towards the body as the prerequisite for an organically continuous rotation between head and trunk as well as the extremities. The physiological rotation of the entire body—due to the neck righting reaction upon passive rotation of the head—in young infants must be replaced by a free rotation between the head and the trunk after the third month of life. Should this not be the case, a deviation could be present. An absent neck righting reaction in a young infant would, upon passive head rotation, give the impression of a free rotation of the head against the trunk and become the expression of a *hypotonic* state. On the other hand, in a 3-month-old infant an en bloc rotation of the entire trunk executed in lieu of a free rotation of the head is a sure sign of the presence of *hypertonicity*.

Balancing Reactions can be examined even in young infants. In most cases the mother's handling of the infant gives hints as to eventual corresponding handicaps. The examination should first be carried out in an abdominal and then in a dorsal position. There should be observation of spontaneous behavior and reactions to handling by the environment, e.g., setting off the Moro reaction (intensity and threshold of arousal).

Counter-reactions by the child are to be expected starting at about 5 months of age for the prone position and at about 6 months of age for the supine position, meaning that the system of balance is better able to adapt to challenges. Tests of sitting, standing on all fours, standing upright, and walking follow. The muscular counter-movements, which take place in normal infants to retain balance upon passive and active changes in position, should be observed intensively. Their absence at a corresponding age can just as well be a sign of the presence of hypotonia with more or less distinct limpness of all muscle groups as it can be a sign of increased but not automatically surmountable muscle tone.

During examination of balance, attention should be paid to the child's behavior. Both overly apprehensive and totally non-apprehensive children should awaken the suspicion of an eventual disturbance in the vestibular system which should then be examined separately. Overburdening always produces anxiety in overly sensitive systems, whereas it produces numbness and, with this, insufficient behavioral reactions in undersensitive systems. Mixtures of both forms are frequently found.

The **tonic patterns of posture** (ATNR, STNR, TLR) present in young infants must fade by 5–6 months of age as their further existence would hamper the increasingly strong appearance of free coordination of movement. The latter is not reliably examinable until this age and can even be detected in pathological cases. In connection with the criteria mentioned above, conclusions can be drawn even in young infants with regard to the persistence to be expected of these tonic patterns of posture from the intensity of the patterns which can be produced. This should at least awaken suspicion and render further examinations necessary.

Asymmetries in posture in young infants that are still under the influence of ATNR are physiologically extant. Suspicion is aroused if they are consistently and irreversibly adopted immediately, again and again, after each change in the child's position. On the other hand, those asymmetries produced through cerebral dominance (the child's favorite position) are interrupted during passive movements and do not return until the child is no longer distracted.

Recognition of **delays in development** naturally requires the child to have reached a certain age at which the manifestation ought to have taken place. Such obvious delays in development in a young infant may be present if it was born prematurely. However, in this case one usually speaks of a child's general immaturity. Categorizing delays in development in young infants often places examiners in the position of having to make difficult decisions. The examiner must know and take into account the entire spectrum of the individual variations of the norm. Nonetheless, it should be possible to voice any suspicion of a delay in development after about 2 months of age and, at least, to call for follow-ups at short intervals. A child who at this age does not make any sounds (the parents should be asked about this), does not in any way react to objects presented to it (e.g., a rattle or bell) and does not smile if enticed to do so almost certainly has a delay in development, most likely even more than that. More important seems to be the partial failure to react, for example, that the child does follow an object with its eyes to the midline and beyond and/or does not show any mimicking or similar reactions whatsoever.

Suspected **disturbances in perceptiveness** in various areas of sensory perception may appear as well. For example, an acute disturbance in perception in spite of intact hearing must be suspected if the child follows a bell with its eyes but shows no reaction if the bell tolls any-where nearby but out of the child's view. The same goes for a situation in which the child overreacts to a noise with uneasiness and screams each time that particular noise can be heard. These disturbances in perception can be recognized early within the first few months of life if adequate aid and quality observation are present.

In summing up, one can say that—individually examined—these criteria for early diagnosis undoubtedly possess different levels of importance. Some, such as the balancing reactions, are not reliably examinable until after 5–6 months of age. However, in their entirety and with due consideration given to the significant individual varia-tions from the norm, they are a valuable indicator of the early diag-nosis of deviations as opposed to normal development. *They should not, however, be rated as an indicator for cerebral motor disturbance or brain damage if they appear as a single finding.*

Over the course of years, each examiner experiences the fact that coordinated or dissociated statomotor delays in development may appear without later developing into a cerebral motor disturbance. During the course of follow-up examinations, some children demon-strate **abnormal cerebral-motor symptoms** which themselves do not yet count as being cerebral motor disturbances but, nevertheless, do call for further regular follow-ups. One single symptom cannot become the expression of such a complex event; it is valued as a warning leading to case-control examinations, which should be continued until all doubts have been eliminated or, if called for, even longer.

Investigations by Other Authors on the Early Diagnosis of Deviations

Early diagnosis has forced itself into our consciousness since the fundamental papers by Köng (1962 a, b, 1965 a, 1972). Starting from normal infant development, the author integrated into her observations her knowledge about primary and/or tonic patterns of posture, which she had observed with regard to their persistence. She was aware of the fact that a disturbed child practices incorrect patterns of movement which are intensified through daily use and which prevent coordination of movement. Using this knowledge as a foundation she developed early diagnosis together with Quinton, which was based upon the work of the Bobaths.

In 1962 she stated that one could never say one was dealing with a "minimal" case after having performed an examination in which obvious symptoms were found. There have been a sufficient number of initially "minimal" cases which—left untreated—developed into severe spastics. We are aware that there are always cases which recede spontaneously; however, there are no methods of differential diagnosis which make it possible to decide which ones those may be. For this reason one should always decide to treat when in doubt. It does not harm the infant if it is treated "for no reason", but it may have terrible consequences for a child's later life if we first observe for a while in order to see how the case develops.

Thirty years later, these statements can only be affirmed. In the meantime, we know that motor capabilities, which may have improved during treatment, do not prove that the remaining sensory integration is not compromised.

We can no longer limit ourselves only to physiotherapy; we must also train physiotherapists to handle extra tasks in the treatment of infants in their first year of life, e.g., tasks of sensory integration. Intensive parental instruction with regard to handling in everyday situations along with the inclusion of specific handling concepts into home life appears to be important.

To Paine (1961, 1964, 1969) the first signs of the presence of a cerebral disturbance of movement at the age of 6–8 months is a lack of smiling in that phase of life. Often one thinks of deafness or blindness of the child when, in reality, it is a central processing disturbance and the sensory organs themselves do not appear to be affected. Changes in postural tone (both increased and decreased) can be found very early. However, these did not become apparent to him until around the 3rd–4th month of life, as did the asymmetries which sometimes can give the impression of a hemiparesis. A decrease in movement during the process of motor development in the early stage of development and abnormal reactions on examination of primary reflexes appear to him to be early signs of motor handicaps.

Milani-Comparetti and Gidoni (1967 a, b) give a limited number of indications which are viewed as early forms of disturbances if they deviate from the norm, namely deviations of: (1) Righting reactions, (2) Parachute reactions, (3) Balancing reactions, and (4) Primitive reactions.

1. Righting reactions

a. Righting reaction of the head, meaning positioning of the head in space

b. Sagittal righting reaction of the trunk with a stretched thorax and stretched hips in a prone position

c. Derotated righting reaction, that is, of the body towards the body, e.g., when the shoulder area turns, the trunk and the hips follow beginning at about the 4th month of life

All of these described reactions are in close relationship to the upright position through the antigravity control of the body's axis (head control, sitting, standing).

2. Parachute reaction

Here, we are dealing with reactions of the extremities to sudden changes of the upright trunk; for example, readiness to jump or stand upon a sudden approach of the arms or legs to the underlying surface. Also belonging to this process is the changing of the body position in space through more or less rapid sideways sloping.

3. Balancing reactions

These reactions appear when the body endeavors to retain balance upon slow or rapid loss of balance. They are subject to the sequences of development.

4. Primitive reflexes (reactions)

The authors believe that it is sensible to call these reactions "primitive" because they are normal very early in life and must disappear during the course of development. Persistence or rapid reaction to the arousal of such responses and, alongside this, the loss of posture control seem to be relevant with regard to early diagnosis.

(These reactions are described in detail beginning on p. 12.)

A development chart, which is primarily oriented around rising up from the unstable horizontal position into the stable vertical position, is added to these views by the authors. It functions so as to make a screening examination possible.

In an in-depth study, S. Sainte-Anne Dargassies (1972) gives comparisons of normal and abnormal development. She subdivides the infants into the following key age-groups:

– Newborns

– 3rd month after birth

– 4th–6th month after birth

– 7th–9th month after birth

– 10th–12th month after birth

and includes examination sheets which place the *psychoaffective* deviations opposite the *motor* ones. Through the system of these examination sheets, she quickly succeeds in obtaining an overall view of the existing disturbances and of how the examiner can judge them or arrive at a prognosis. The author's goal is to achieve as complete an overview as possible of the deviations in development with the option of comparing previous examination notes with current ones.

Touwen (1975) examined a large number of children for 1½ years with regard to the appearance and disappearance of reactions and patterns of development and completed a set of statistics on a number of important items.

According to von Bernuth (1972), early diagnosis during the course of the first year of life rests upon (1) judging general findings, (2) general developmental diagnostics, and (3) the actual neurological examination.

From the multitude of general findings which one comes across continuously in infants with cerebral damage, some should be emphasized:

● Intense startle reaction

● Frequent crying without cause

● Disturbances in sleeping-waking rhythm

● Drinking difficulties

● Hypersalivation

● Marbled skin

These nonspecific symptoms—along with other pathological indications—can be important indicators of damage.

Dubowitz (1983) suggests that when dealing with newborns displaying conspicuous signs, particular attention should be paid to noting whether or not the infant is able to overcome these difficulties or whether they remain.

In addition to the neurological examination, which is not always satisfactory, it is now possible to determine the type and precise location of the anatomic lesion through cranial sonography, computed tomography, magnetic resonance imaging (MRI), evoked potentials, electroencephalography, and velocity of nerve conduction. Hearing and vision tests make it possible to determine neuronal deficits and to compare them with graphic techniques.

Dubowitz labels this mode of action the "integrated way of thinking." It gives very precise indications for the neurological examination and shows various states related to a multitude of different disturbances which differ particularly in the severity of the illness. This is demonstrated by using as an example asphyxia or intraventricular bleeding. The technique used in this examination is precisely explained in the paper. The author employs an examination form based on her own experience and that of other authors such as Brazelton (1973), Amiel-Tison (1968), Prechtl (1977), Parmelee and Michaelis (1971), and Sainte-Anne Dargassies (1977).

She believes that with the help of her integrated way of thinking, it will be possible to establish a foundation for future follow-up examinations and for prognosis, in addition to grounds for action by the physician in cases of lack of oxygen or cerebral hemorrhaging in the newborn.

Casaer and Eggermont (1983) investigated similar aspects. They believe that risk assessment for future developmental abnormalities cannot be founded on only one factor, rather a thorough case history of all occurrences up to the date of the examination should be compiled. For this purpose, they recommend using the optimum score scale according to Prechtl (1977). Furthermore, they suggest recording all events that take place in the newborn and intensive-care wards, a description of behavioral states according to Prechtl (1968) and Michaelis et al. (1979), as well as noting the infant's behavior while breathing and being fed. Data such as body size and head circumference should be recorded. Reports by the nursing staff should also be considered.

Neurosensory functions are registered using a diagnosis form that was compiled based on the author's own experience as well as that of the above-mentioned authors and others (such as André-Thomas and colleagues 1960; Dubowitz 1985, Parmelee and Schulte 1970, Touwen 1978).

Following critical analysis of these examination steps, the decision is made as to whether the child merely requires regular check-ups to keep the situation under control or whether treatment must be initiated accordingly.

Causes of Cerebral Palsy

Cerebral palsy is the result of lesions or malformations of the central nervous system. Except in cases of hereditary familial genetic defects, these injuries occur pre-, peri-, or postnatally. In 20–30% of all pregnancies, there are risk factors for the fetus (Dudenhausen and Saling, 1967).

Currently, 10–15% of all newborns are not born under "optimum conditions" (Schröter, 1967). The gravest threat to the fetus and the newborn is a depleted oxygen supply. Even a brief lack of oxygen can lead to permanent organ damage. This holds particularly true for the brain. Up until 1967, risk indices were compiled according to a so-called "nonoptimal score" on the assumption that this would not only improve information on the causes of handicaps, but also put specialists into a position to sort out those infants in greatest need of special surveillance, such as follow-up examinations. After it became obvious that this method was leaving the examiners with such an impossibly large number of children to follow, Prechtl (1968) advanced the idea of developing an "optimum score" index. It was later modified by Michaelis.

This index contains 42 items which provide for optimum conditions for pregnancy and birth. These are optimal requirements which must be fulfilled by the mother during pregnancy and by the child before and during birth. A quantitative neurological study of 1378 newborns was carried out during their first 10 days of life and statistically validated through correlation analysis with the pregnancy and delivery data as well as the child's condition after birth.

The 42 variables pertaining to pre- and perinatal history were analysed and estimated in order to find out to what extent they deviated from the optimum. Thus, an obstetrical risk score was calculated for each child. The further the conditions deviated from the norm, the larger was the number of related nonoptimal conditions. By simply adding up the number of nonoptimal conditions, it became possible to pick out those infants who ran the risk of having neurological damage.

Prechtl's examination led to the following assessment:

– Low-risk group: 0–1 nonoptimal item (19.2%)

– Medium-risk group: 2–6 nonoptimal items (68.4%)

– High-risk group: 7 or more nonoptimal items (12.4%)

If one decides to work with the optimum risk method as in Prechtl's index, one obtains good information about the amount of risk the child incurred. For example, Prechtl found that among the high-risk children, many weighed less than 2,500 g at birth and also showed signs of an apathy syndrome. Children with hemisyndromes, for example, were found in all three groups, while children with the hyperexcitability syndrome were most numerous in the medium-risk group. Statistics show that there were more boys in this group than girls.

Criteria for optimal obstetrical conditions (Prechtl, 1965)

1)	Mother's age (primipara)	18−30 years
	Mother's age (multipara)	20−30 years
2)	Mother's legal status	married
3)	Number of births	1−6
4)	Previous miscarriages	0−2
5)	Pelvis	no disproportion
6)	Luetic infections	absent
7)	Rh-antagonism	absent
8)	Blood-group incompatibility	absent
9)	Nutritional status	good
10)	Hemoglobin level	70% or above (> 8 g%)
11)	Pregnancy hemorrhaging	absent
12)	Infections during pregnancy	absent
13)	Abdominal X-ray examinations during pregnancy	none
14)	Toxemia of pregnancy	absent or mild
15)	Blood pressure	not significantly over or under 135/90
16)	Albuminuria or edema	absent
17)	Hyperemesis	absent
18)	Emotional stress	absent
19)	Involuntary infertility (2 years)	absent
20)	Chronic illness in the mother	absent

Birth

21)	Twins or multiple births	none
22)	Delivery	spontaneous
23)	Length of first stage	6−24 h
24)	Length of second stage	10 min to 2 h
25)	Labor pains	medium or strong
26)	Medication for the mother	Oxygen, local anesthesia
27)	Amniotic fluid	clear
28)	Rupture of the amnion	no more than 6 h

Fetal factors

29)	Intrauterine position	vertex
30)	Gestational age	38−41 weeks
31)	Fetal presentation	vertex
32)	Cardiac action	regular
33)	Heart rate (2nd stage)	100−160
34)	Twist in umbilical cord	none or loose
35)	Prolapse of the umbilical cord	none
36)	Knots in the umbilical cord	none
37)	Placental infarction	none or small
38)	Onset of breathing	during the first minute
39)	Treatment, resuscitation	none

40) Medication given	none
41) Body temperature	normal
42) Birth weight	2,500−4,990 g

These criteria for optimal obstetrical conditions now need to be revised. According to Touwen (personal communication), Prechtl and his colleagues used an optimal score index containing 73 items. A statistical reappraisal of the changed items has not taken place to date. It is the obligation of the peri- or neonatologist to work out a new optimal score index.

The principle of this type of risk index is the reason for citing it at this point, although the number and choice of the items are not in accordance with today's obstetrical demands. Each item is given a score of 0 or 1; the latter is given if the result is not optimal. This optimal score scala is a suggested method for selecting children born with medium to high risk factors. This group as well as children who show conspicuous neurological signs during the period following birth constitute those in need of careful follow-up examinations.

A final revision was carried out in 1979 by Michaelis et al. and a new list of further optimal conditions was compiled.

A reduction in optimality of child development can be expected wherever conspicuous maternal findings in the anamnesis have been found. Premature births and miscarriages in the mother's medical history as well as bleeding during the first trimester, early labor, surgical deliveries, and premature births combined with Apgar Scores less than 7 all show correlation with abnormal findings in the children at a later date.

Children to be included with the ones showing conspicuous neurological findings during the period after birth are those with the following behavioral syndromes (Prechtl, 1968; Schulte, 1968):

- Apathy syndrome
- Hemisyndrome
- Hypertonia syndrome
- Hyperexcitability syndrome
- Hypotonia syndrome

The reader will find a detailed description of the syndromes in the diagnostic section of this book. They complete the risk factor index. Further risk factors can be found in postnatal illnesses which bring about disturbances in brain function. First and foremost are meningo-encephalitides and/or encephalitides of diverse etiologies (both viral and bacterial origin) and severe nutritional disturbances. The large number of children injured in traffic accidents also carry a major risk following brain injuries. Extensive social deprivation with neglect and lack of stimulation produces high developmental risks as well.

A smaller number of children are born with obvious defects. Belonging to this group are children suffering from a chromosome aberration (e.g., the Down syndrome) as well as children with deformities that can affect part of the central nervous system (e.g., schistases such as spina bifida and congenital hydrocephalus). Enzymatic defects are the cause of a variety of brain functional disturbances (e.g., phenylketonuria, galactosemia). These children should be examined at regular intervals beginning at birth in order to develop necessary methods of treatment when needed.

In summary, the following factors are considered to be the cause of motor disabilities:

1. Inappropriate locomotor experience (e.g., spasticity, athetosis, ataxia and its mixed forms)

2. Inappropriate or inadequate locomotor experience combined with tactile-kinesthetic, optical, and acoustic perceptual disorders

3. Inadequate locomotor experience (as in cases of social deprivation and mental retardation)

4. Psychologically caused disturbances of locomotor experience

5. Genetically caused disturbances of locomotor experience

6. Mixed forms of the above

Examination Technique

Early diagnosis depends heavily on the observation of abnormal co-ordination of posture and movement. Knowledge of normal locomotor development is the fundamental prerequisite for such evaluation. The younger the infant, the more the examination results fluctuate, under certain circumstances even on the same day. Furthermore, there are dynamic phases in locomotor development during the first year of life in which one must expect to find varying results. One must not overlook the multitude of variations within locomotor development which are often not sufficiently taken into account.

As a means of obtaining as exact and as reliable results as possible —despite these difficulties— it is important to create a constant environment for the examination. In order to make certain that nothing of importance is overlooked and to ensure consistency of follow-up examinations, one should stick to a fixed order of examination steps. Furthermore, it is necessary to document the child's condition at each examination. The "states" of Prechtl and Beintema have proven to be useful here.

The expression "states"—understood as being the child's condition, for example, its degree of awareness—was defined by Ashby (1956): "One defines the condition of the state of 'a system' as each well-defined requirement or characteristic that is discernible if it recurs continuously."

Prechtl and Beintema (1964) describe the following six criteria:

State 1: Eyes closed, no movement
State 2: Eyes closed, irregular breathing, no simple movement
State 3: Eyes opened, no gross movements
State 4: Eyes opened, some gross movements, no crying
State 5: Eyes opened or closed, crying
State 6: Other findings/syndromes which should be described (e.g., coma)

Objective criteria are not dealt with here but rather heterogeneous combinations of varying quality such as breathing, motor activity, open or closed eyelids. The authors consider it possible that other variables exist; however, at the same time, they believe these criteria to be the easiest to recognize. Three examiners, who looked at a total of 80 children, all gave an identical judgement on the states.

What appears to be ideal if the examiner succeeds in keeping the child in state 4. This is not always possible. Most important is to document each change. Factors having to do with the child's internal environment and daily rhythm, etc. are not to be excluded. By "constant" environment we mean that the examinations should be carried out under identical conditions each time.

As in the examination of newborns, one should examine the baby that has been brought in by its mother or guardian in a calm, quiet atmosphere. Any type of disruption from outside (such as a telephone) should be avoided. The room should be warm, but not overheated. There should be diffuse light as the child otherwise turns toward the light, thereby giving the impression that asymmetries may be present.

A child that is hungry or has just been woken up is difficult to examine.

It is recommended to spend the first 10 min observing the child as it sits in its mother's lap during which time one can discuss the child's case history.

It has been shown that a child whose mother trusts the examiner is quiet from the beginning of the examination. A mother who is not trusting or is apprehensive will transfer her own anxiety to the child.

An overly sensitive vestibular system will cause the mother to carry out all movements with the infant both slowly and very close to the mother. Since these sensitive children cry a lot, observing the mother's handling with regard to attempts to pacify the child (e.g. by rocking it in either a vertical or horizontal position) is informative.

While undressing the child lying on its back, there is frequently an intensive Moro reaction upon which the child cries even more. Hence, the dorsal position becomes an unpleasant experience and strongly irritates child, mother, and examiner. Dressing and undressing, therefore, turns into an event that is carried out reluctantly.

The child is undressed by the mother and placed naked and in a **supine position** onto the examining table. This has proven to be the most useful position as an infant generally does not like being put back into the dorsal position later in the course of the examination.

The examiner tries to come into contact with the child through glances and language without touching it. The child's spontaneous motor response and posture become best recognizable as well as assessable this way (motoscopy).

By using toys or eye contact, one tries to stimulate the child to move its head from one side to the other. All the while the examiner observes shoulder placement and the movement of the arms, trunk, hips, and legs. Depending upon the child's age, one attempts to stimulate it to grasp for an object which is being held in front of its eyes at a distance that it can reach.

If the child does not spontaneously grab the object, the examiner touchs the child's hand lightly with the object and observes whether the child then reaches for it. The examiner also tries to learn to what extent the child is capable of seizing objects at midline or even beyond it. The examiner should particularly observe the placing of arms and hands to determine whether they are in supination or pronation. The manner of grasping must also be observed as must the placing of hips, legs, and feet and their movements.

In order to avoid a hyperexcitable reaction during the examination it is often useful to perform it with the child on its mother's lap. The child should sit up straight with its back leaning against the mother's stomach. The mother should not touch her child. The examiner sits in front of mother and child and slightly pulls the child's legs at the calves in order to bring it into a lying position.

In a hyperexcitable child the examiner will note that it opens its eyes widely or its mouth or that its hands and arms take on an extended position, similar to the beginning of a Moro reaction. If these signals take place very distinctly and rapidly, one can speak of an overly extensive vestibular reaction upon change of position. The movements and handling of the child should be carried out calmly and slowly, because otherwise it will soon begin to cry.

The next step is turning the child over into the **prone position** in order to find out whether or not it is capable of surmounting the physiological flexion tonus of the first few months of life, of raising its head and bringing its arms to the front on its own. A child that is spontaneously willing to turn over should not be touched, but rather be stimulated into turning over on its own through "social contact" (e.g. a smile from the examiner, noises, toys, etc.). The type of rotation should be closely observed. The child should be allowed to rotate to the right as well as to the left. Leg and hip placement should be taken note of during the course of rotation as well as in the prone position. Special attention should be paid to the head placement while the child is in an asymmetrical position. The examiner should stimulate the child with toys or noises into a change of position so as to determine whether the asymmetrical position is fixed or can be overcome spontaneously.

As soon as the child has turned onto its back again, it is made to sit by means of traction while paying particular attention to head control. Afterwards, the child's ability to support itself while sitting is tested in a forward, sideways, and backward position. The child's readiness to stand is observed by having its legs rapidly approach the underlying surface whereas observing the child's readiness to jump is accomplished by having its arms quickly approach the underlying surface. Finally, older children are tested for their ability to sit while balancing themselves, crawl, stand, and walk. The following prerequisites are necessary for this: head control, ability to rotate around the body axis, and development of the balancing/static reaction.

Not only the observation of the motor behavior gives information about deviations, the capability of the child to involve itself in an interaction with the examiner is important. The child's eventual irritability or its capability to adapt to a new situation are significant criteria for determining the state of health of its nervous system.

The following chapters contain the examination steps which are most favorable in each individual case while taking into consideration the level of development to be expected in the specified month of life. This is done at monthly intervals from months 1 through 10 and, after that, only in months 12, 15, and 18. Partially, the system of gradation is based on the Denver Scales of Development (which correspond to the Gesell Scales) in order to establish an easily remembered, consistent system to refer to for the individual examination steps.

Sequence of Examination Steps for the Neurological Motoscopic Examination of Infants

A. Case history by the parents including reference to all documents available from previous examinations and hospital treatments. In some cases, family photographs may also be useful.

B. Neurological examinations with consideration given to gestational age, particularly when examining very small infants.

C. Motoscopic examination of coordinated movements (eventually aided by external stimulation such as toys, eye contact, etc.).

D. Observations of behavior with consideration of dynamics, ability to adapt, irritability, motion in space, sensitivity to touch (tactility and proprioception).

The examination should take place in the following sequence (according to age):

Gross motor ability

- Supine position
- Prone position
- Raising up from the supine position
- Attaining and holding a standing position with support under the arms
- Pulling upward to a sitting position
- Sitting down unaided
- Sitting
- Pulling upward to a standing position
- Standing up unaided
- Standing
- Rolling, creeping
- Crawling
- Walking
- Posture and muscle tone
- Test of postural reflexes in all positions (horizontal and head-down position, lateral displacement, etc.)

- Reactions of balance
- Symmetry
- Tonic postural patterns and reflexes as well as reactions of early infancy (primary reactions)

Fine motor function and adaption
Grasping
Speech and social contact

- Speech
- Social contact

Hearing and localizing noises
Phonation while watching breathing, sucking, and swallowing

Vision and eye movements
Routines of daily life
Emotional behavior
Development (with consideration of sensory integration)

- Visual
- Acoustic
- Tactile-kinesthetic-vestibular

In summing up, one can say that in order to recognize deviations in an infant's development, knowledge of the normal course of development is imperative. Along with the criteria already mentioned that signal deviations, Sainte-Anne Dargassies (1972) considered the following.

While examining, several main principles should be kept in mind:

1. The maturation process is continuous. It is a dynamic developmental process. Any disruption in or lack of continuous development should, in itself, already be considered as a suspicious sign.

2. Upon this foundation of acquisition of capabilities, the psychoaffective functions, which appear during the course of the first 6 months of life, must be observed. After this age, motor function while in the upright position is of major significance. More important than the point in time of the mere appearance of these capabilities, however, is their quality and the way they influence play.

3. It is important to understand which components make up the child's behavior, whether the motor or the psychoaffective component is being dealt with. Observation must include both the current condition as well as the degree of maturation achieved since birth.

A single examination does not yield conclusive information as to the state of development. Follow-up examinations provide data for prognosis. For this reason, Sainte-Anne Dargassies has selected the third, eighth, and tenth months of age as "key" ages. We prefer the follow-up timetable mentioned in the preventative medicine pamphlet (3rd–10th day; 4th–6th week; 6th–7th month; 10th–12th month, etc.) since early treatment should begin before the fifth month.

Statements made too hastily regarding a child's condition can lead to a feeling of distrust about the examiner's precision and does not contribute to the relaxing family atmosphere so vital to the child.

Initial conspicuous signs may be distinguishable through motor indications, although their full complexity may not become apparent until a much later date.

The following is an example of an observation that can be made very easily in small infants and which can often have far-reaching consequences. While performing a traction test from the supine position on an approximately 4-month-old infant with motor deviations, the head usually hangs down toward the back while the child is extended. The mouth can be open during each extension. In some cases, no eye contact with the mother takes place (Figs. **17, 18**). Soon thereafter, the child demonstrates drinking and eating difficulties which may seriously impair the mother-child contact. The lack of eye contact sometimes aggravates this problem until it becomes truly unbearable.

Consequently, it is not surprising that the child demonstrates eating and speech disturbances later on. As a result, the child develops behavioral disturbances, which appear to be conspicuous, caused by the mother's unintentionally false behavior that, in itself, had merely adapted to the given situation. Such conspicuous child behavior often leads to a visit to the doctor's office. Should the examiner misinterpret the mother's behavior by not giving substantial consideration to the background of the individual case, this type of situation sometimes becomes even more aggravated. In this manner, motor deviations may lead to serious disturbances at a very early age should they not be recognized in time and treated methodically.

More explicit knowledge about the early signs of motor deviations, including visual, acoustic, and tactile-kinesthetic integration as well as continuously improving methods of treatment will allow us to comprehend better the issue of multiple handicaps in children. We have at present merely scratched the surface.

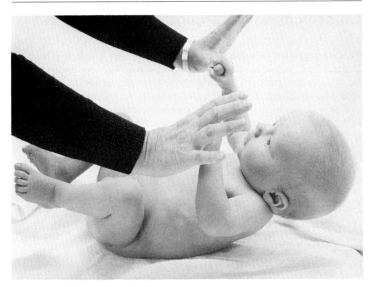

Fig. **17**

Fig. **18**

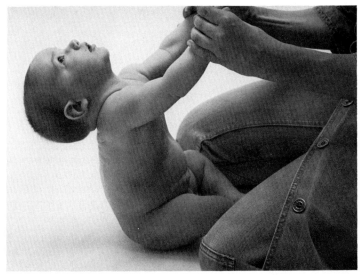

Classification of Cerebral Palsy

Despite numerous studies carried out by various research groups, it has not been possible to come up with a generally accepted definition for the characteristics of cerebral palsy. Contrary to adult neurological illnesses, which are based on pathologically and anatomically clearly outlined characteristics and corresponding, definable disturbed functions, the noxious agent of infantile brain injury, e.g., lack of oxygen, diffusely affects the still completely immature brain in an unpredictable manner and with various degrees of intensity. Due to the fact that the process of compensation produced by the brain (the brain has a considerable amount of "plasticity" at that age) may balance out a portion of the disturbed function, the result is unpredictable, and manifold pathological features appear.

As long as light has not been shed on the course of individual neuropathological events—to date, only hypotheses have been put forth which involve more or less high probabilities—any endeavor to categorize must restrict itself to very precise descriptions and distinguishing boundaries of the characteristic features belonging to the symptoms of infantile brain damage.

According to Perlstein (1952), hardly any two human beings with cerebral palsy are alike with regard to the prominent features and the severity of their illness. Nonetheless, he considers a classification attempt to be useful. He proposes four groups:

1. Spasticity
2. Hyperkinesis
   - Athetosis
   - Dystonia
   - Tremor
3. Rigidity
4. Ataxia

A definition of the general term cerebral palsy was worded as follows in 1959 after a lengthy discussion by the *Oxford Study Group on Child Neurology and Cerebral Palsy:* Cerebral palsy is a disturbance of both the child's posture as well as its movement. It is a non-progressive ailment which is acquired during early development.

In its fully developed stage, this motor disturbance is divided into 5 different types; nevertheless, it is the mixed forms which occur most frequently:

A Spasticity
- Quadruplegia
- Diparesis
- Hemiparesis
- Bilateral hemiparesis

B Athetosis
- Dystonic form
- Choreoathetotic form
- Rigid form

C Ataxia

D Central hypotonia

E Mixed forms

A Spasticity

One of the main chacteristics of spasticity is muscle hypertonicity, which results in poor coordination of movement and poor sustainment of posture. In order to carry out a movement in a coordinated manner, the level of both the agonists and the antagonists must be adequately regulated, a function which is no longer possible if a brain lesion has occurred.

In the case of spasticity there is only limited mobility, to which the central control mechanism attempts to adapt. Tonic postural patterns prevent coordination. Stereotyped movements as well as depletion of possibilites for movement appear: The extremities become stiff.

The term "quadruplegia" means that all four extremities and, with them, the entire body, are equally affected.

The term "diparesis" implies that the legs are more strongly affected than the upper extremities.

The term "hemiparesis" characterizes spasticity of only one side of the body, while the other side demonstrates normal tone quality in the extremities.

Finally, in the case of "bilateral hemiparesis" one side of the body is strongly affected and the other, only slightly. Despite the fact that all four extremities are part of the clinical picture in this case, the term "quadruplegia" would be inappropriate due to the varying degrees of intensity of the spasticity.

B Athetosis

Whereas spasticity leads to a decline in a child's movements, athetosis is more of an oversteering within the locomotor system.

Hence, the afflicted children continuously perform undirected, useless, and—to the observer—quite frequently bizarre-looking movements. The lack of meaningful, economical coordination of movement is obvious. The child does not seem able to take on a fixed position. The more intensely the child willfully attempts to do so,. the less successful it is.

C Ataxia

In cases of ataxia, the feedback mechanism of the central regulating system has been damaged by disturbances of the movement control apparatus of the cerebellum and its nerve tracts. Permanent co-contraction, which is also an expression of oversteering in the central nervous system, is the result. Therefore, ataxia and athetosis have very similar phenotypes. A large number of athetotics simultaneously demonstrate ataxic signs and symptoms. The oversteering results in a lack of coordination of movement as in athetosis. There is a lack of balance. Children with athetosis help themselves by using a postural attitude which can also facilitate maintenance of balance at a later age.

When these children begin to walk, they do so with the "stilted" stride so typical in cases of ataxia, while the upper extremities demonstrate patterns of extension. As a result of an intention tremor, fine motor movements and manipulations frequently cannot be carried out in a coordinated manner.

D Central Hypotonia

When dealing with central hypotonia, coordinated regulation seems completely impossible. The control mechanism is at a complete standstill. Movements that are carried out despite this happen with such roughness and abruptness that they produce extreme effects. Attaining as well as maintaining posture become impossible. All attempts are frustrating. After a while, the child gives up and remains lying quietly, sometimes even listlessly, on its back or stomach. In the horizontal position the child sometimes develops quite a considerable feeling for balance during the course of its general development; however, all attempts to raise itself against the pull of gravity fail. Some children occasionally only demonstrate their inability to attain intermediate stages of movement when in an upright position.

Also belonging to this group of conspicuous signs are tactile-kinesthetic-vestibular disturbances of perception.

E Mixed Forms

Mixed forms are more difficult to identify. These are also the most commonly found forms in children with motor disturbances. They exhibit faulty coordination of movement.

Here, it must be pointed out that the motor disturbance is only part of the overall injury. In almost all cases—with various degrees of intensity—the afflicted individual suffers from multiple handicaps. The motor disturbance is merely the most obvious aspect. However, it only represents the tip of the iceberg. It frequently takes a considerable amount of time to localize further damage. Above all, during the first year of life, motor disturbance is—in most cases—given prominence since, at this age, it is the foundation for perception, recognition, and the capability of utilizing integrated sensory organs.

The degree of disability of differentiated child performance or perception cannot be demonstrated and diagnosed until the developmental prerequisites have appeared.

Milani-Comparetti and Gidoni see the dynamic process of development of the structure of posture and movement in infants all the way up to the upright walking child as an interaction of "competing patterns" that come and go and are built in during the course of the developmental process. Delayed development with regard to the milestones and the appearance of abnormal patterns of posture and movement are to them the fundamental signs for early recognition of cerebral palsy.

These characteristic, abnormal patterns of posture and movement can be recorded by a so-called motoscopy as neurologists have been doing for some time when dealing with cases of athetosis and ataxia. In particular, these two clinical pictures could never be completely explained by muscle tone alone. Spasticity, dystonia, and rigidity were also evaluated through a motoscopic examination and then divided into two characteristic groups:

A. Characteristic pattern with extension. The lower extremities are extended and adducted, inwardly rotated, and crossed. The upper extremities show shoulder retraction, flexed elbows, and hand joints. Under other circumstances, a complete flexion pattern is present.

B. Characterized by extension without adduction of the lower extremities; not crossed. The feet are inwardly rotated, the upper extremities are bent at the shoulder, the elbows stretched, and the arms rotated toward the inside.

Group A consists mainly of spastics and group B, mainly of children with dystonic disturbances.

Nonetheless, even motoscopic examination alone should not be used as the ultimate way to judge a child's condition. A multitude of parameters produce a mosaic picture.

Discovering deviations from normal development during the period following birth—especially with regard to establishing a prognosis—is exceedingly difficult. Prechtl and Beintema elaborated on reflexes and reactions according to standardized studies of 1500 newborns whose mothers had shown conspicuous signs during pregnancy. This elaboration is designed to simplify recognition of conspicuous neurological signs.

This clinical neurological examination put the authors into a position to *quantify* syndromes. Prechtl and Schulte distinguished between the following syndromes, which made way for more explicit judgement of the child's state with regard to the basic disorder and allowed for the introduction of suitable measures:

1. Hyperexcitability Syndrome

This syndrome is found in children with exaggerated proprioceptive and externally evoked reactions. In some cases, clonus appears which is not quickly exhausted. The child's Moro reaction overshoots the usual extent. Sometimes it is not even necessary for the examiner to arouse this reaction, because it happens at the slightest movement of the head.

The child responds to a touch or sudden, faint noise with an exaggerated reaction. These children cry a lot and sleep little. Following a clinical examination without any abnormal findings, the prognosis for such overly excitable children is good. Check-ups show, however, that these children remain restless to a certain degree and are easily aroused by outside stimuli.

Some hyperkinetic, hyperactive children have a hyperexcitable syndrome in their history which is sometimes linked with disturbances in concentration as well as distractability, which can cause learning problems.

2. Apathy Syndrome

The opposite of overly excitable children is the one that is extremely quiet and listless. Proprioceptive and externally evoked reactions are sluggish and difficult to stimulate. Stepping, Galant, Bauer, grasping, and Moro reactions can only be elicited with difficulty, if at all.

When these children cry, it sounds like a quiet, continuous wail. They require lots of sleep and either have difficulties with or cannot swallow at all, meaning that they must often be tube fed. The prognosis for these children without clinical examination and treatment is not good. In this case, we are faced with a more or less severe impairment of the nervous system.

3. Muscle Hypertonia

Here, we are dealing with increased resistance to passive movements; however, fully fledged flexion and extension patterns can still be noted in their posture. All joints seem immovable, unable to be flexed or extended. When the child moves, it does so only in its entirety. In most cases, active movement is limited. Hypertonia may be more severe in either the lower or upper extremities. When raising the child upward, its arms are tightly bent. Due to the fact that as hypertonia exists in newborns physiologically, differentiation is sometimes difficult and frequently depends upon the examiner's experience.

4. Muscle Hypotonia

If all proprioceptive and external reactions can be stimulated in a case of hypotonia, it may be assumed that the syndrome is of cerebral origin. The child's arms are limply extended when raised; the child lies down nearly flat on the underlying surface in a frog-like position. The reactions for overcoming gravity are not good. At times, the child either moves its body very little or too much, because it constantly over-compensates for its floppy tone, hence appearing to be restless. These children sometimes, for example, raise their heads up while lying in a prone position. This movement, however, is greatly exaggerated. At times, the child lays its head on one side but extends it backward very far. When examined passively, the joints seem to be overextendible. All positions are unstable. The prognosis, when dealing with hypotonia, depends on the cause of the condition.

5. Hemisyndrome

Upon detailed clinical observation, asymmetrical reactions are repeatedly noted. This aspect is characterized by little or no movement on one side or by asymmetrical reactions (e.g., Moro reaction). The range of neurological examinations should be expanded to include explicit observation of movement.

In 1964, a small group of investigators in Edinburgh attempted to work out a terminology and classification of cerebral palsy. For reasons already given, they concluded that it is actually only possible to speak of a "syndrome of cerebral dysfunction" in the broadest sense of the word. Excluded from this study were all neurogenic and muscular illnesses of the motor apparatus as well as those which appear for only a short period and are most likely of psychological origin, all progres-

sive neurological disturbances as well as those neurological disturbances seen in mentally retarded children. The authors believed that
classification would only be possible when better knowledge about the
etiologic causes of cerebral motor disturbances had been attained.
However, 11 years later, Hagberg published his classification of cerebral motor disturbances mainly based on the observation and interpretation of clinical features. He distinguished the following:

● Spasticity syndrome, including hemiplegia, diparesis, and spastic
  quadruplegia

● Ataxia syndrome, including two variations: congenital ataxia and
  ataxic diparesis

● Dyskinesia with hyperkinesia in cases of the choreoathetoid form
  and the dystonic form

● Mixed forms

The term "cerebral motor disturbance" first appears in German literature in 1965 in a work by Köng. It is used instead of the term "cerebral palsy" since it is in actual fact *not a paralysis*—which means
decreased muscle power—but rather a *sensorimotor disturbance of coordination*. The author considers this term better for psychological
reasons so as not to burden less affected cases with such a severe
sounding expression. This term has the further advantage of being
more precise, as neither a paresis nor a paralysis is present here.

According to Milani-Comparetti (1964), the neurological explanation
for comprehending patterns of posture and movement is a question of
the regulation of precisely these patterns over the subordinate mechanisms of muscle tension. Hence, it becomes possible to explain the fact
that the primary aspect pertaining to cerebral motor disturbance is a
brain lesion which causes a disturbance in the structure of the motor
functioning patterns and, secondly, leads to a change in muscle tone
which does not become manifest until later. Thus, it is better to speak
of disturbances of posture and movement than to speak of spasticity,
rigidity, dystonia, hypertonia, or hypotonia.

In cases of cerebral motor disturbances, the abnormal patterns are the
central issue. These range from total lack of posture in a listless child to
excessive tone in a stiff, spastic child whose movements are limited,
hence giving the impression of a paresis.

According to Sherrington (1964), the tone of a muscle is unimportant
with regard to the ailment itself. It is only significant when considering
its distribution among all of the body's muscles with respect to the
child's pattern of posture. The interaction of gravity and muscle tone
yields patterns of posture and movement which are needed by every

individual in order to have the capability of starting or of arresting movement.

If it is assumed by Milani-Comparetti (1964) that with cerebral motor disturbance one is dealing with a neurological ailment, the neurologist should bear in mind that posture and movement of the body are the result of operational decisions made by the central nervous system and can, therefore, be interpreted as the integration of patterns of movement independent of the mechnics of such processes. Milani-Comparetti suggests a motoscopic classification of cerebral palsy which seems to be more useful than the nomenclature, which is tone oriented (Table **3**).

Jackson (1958) expresses this with the following succinct sentence: "The brain knows no muscles; it knows only movement."

Table **3** Motoscopic classification of cerebral motor disturbances

Lack of postural control	(Delayed motor development = delay in development of primary automatisms against the force of gravitiy; this is traditionally called the image of the "floppy child" or "hypotonic child"). It can be observed in both normal and mentally handicapped children. It can, however, be an early phase of development or a partial aspect of cerebral palsy whose typical patterns are still recognizable despite the sparse drive of motor ability and postural attitude. The later the final stage of cerebral palsy appears, the more severe the mental handicap is.		
Regression syndrome (dominance of fetal patterns)	**I. Diarchy** (Greek: dual rule)		In cases which are not adequately treated, a functional compromise later develops between the two dominant patterns, this compromise being total semi-flexion. The syndrome may be tetra-, para-, or hemiparetic, although it occurs mainly in the lower extremities. It is accompanied by spasticity.
	Extension pattern Upper extremities: retracted shoulders, bent elbows, bent wrist including ulnar deviation, closed fist, adducted thumb Lower extremities: extended, adducted, inwardly rotated (crossed)	**Bending pattern** Upper and lower extremities totally bent	

Table 3   (continued)

II. Diarchy

"Pseudo-Moro" (startle reaction pattern in the supine position on firm surface: arms are abducted, hands curled to claws, forced inhalation, startled facial expression) Lower extremities slightly abducted, feet supinated	**Propulsion** (= pattern of movement carried out by the fetus in order to be born. Fetal cooperation during birth) Trunk is bent forward. One finds the shoulders protracted, the arms flexed and inwardly rotated, the elbows extended and in pronation, bent wrists and hands drawn to fists in the upper extremities with the head extended.	Here, the findings are more severe with regard to the upper extremities and head. Also belonging to the syndrome are dysphagia (disturbances of chewing and swallowing as well as salivation) and dysarthria (tongue movement is limited to the sucking pattern). The missing sideways movement of the tongue leads to the typical deformity of the cavity of the mouth. When the child is preoccupied, especially during propulsion, one can note an opening spasm and disturbances of conjugated eye movements, especially regarding the limitation of downward glance.

Dystonic-athetoid syndromes (uncoordinated integration of the patterns)	The clinical picture is characterized by a disturbance of muscle integration which is the result of a conflict between the patterns. For example, the hand being between not reaching and actually reaching or — when looking at facial expressions — between the pattern which appears upon having tasted something sour or bitter and many others. Particularly typical is the participation of the arm's extension-pronation pattern and the so-called asymmetrical tonic neck reflex. The patterns of the second diarchy may also be a part of the dystonic-athetoid conflict. The corresponding clinical picture is very diverse: it disappears while sleeping, changes as time passes, and, frequently, lack of posture control precedes it.
Ataxic picture	"Dyschronometry". Temporal integration of normal pattern is disturbed (not often recognizable on photographs and usually not diagnosable during the first year of life).

Mixed forms

* (excerpt from MILANI-COMPARETTI, A.: Therapy for neuromotor disturbances in children. In: **Bonavita,** V. Terapia in neurologia)

Treatment of Cerebral Motor Disturbances and Other Deviations

If a normal child is to raise itself up from a horizontal into a vertical position during the course of the first year of life, integration of posture and movement patterns are needed in order to succeed against the force of gravity. The child becomes more and more independent and frees itself of its mother's and other persons' handling within its environment during the course of its development.

Faulty development of these patterns of movement produces abnormal sequences of actions to which the child accustoms itself and which prevent it from fulfilling its desire to move and eventually to achieve the upright position. These faulty sequences prevent normal development in a broad sense.

Development of voluntary patterns of movement occurs progressively and in an interlocked fashion, meaning that a certain movement and, subsequently, maintaining that position is built up upon already existing features in an overlapping manner. No intermediate stages are omitted from this development. In order to allow an upright position to be attained against the force of gravity, muscle tone must develop sufficiently to be strong and differentiated enough to overcome gravity and simultaneously allow for the performance of more refined movements.

In addition, there are reflex mechanisms which regulate maintenance of the upright position, balance, and posture during the course of the sequences of movement. A normal posture reflex mechanism guarantees normal posture tone and allows for normal patterns of movement. One of the first retaining reactions for which normal posture tone is a prerequisite is head control.

Within the first few months, the infant begins to develop the physiological flexion tone learned in utero into stretching and, further still, into raising of its head. Thus, the body extension in the prone position with raising of the head against the force of gravity begins and is completed at about 6 months of age upon full extension from the hip, after which higher grade, more differentiated retaining reactions, such as balancing and body righting reactions, follow. These must be prepared so as to assure that rotation and supporting reactions come into effect.

Exact knowledge of a child's motor function, including integration of perceptive functions, makes it possible to draw up a treatment plan, always orientated to the child's signals. Hence, before treatment may be commenced, the therapist should perform tests of function in order to be able to judge the goal of treatment and the steps needed to achieve this:

● Observation of motor development taking age into consideration.

● Examination of motor functions, such as head control, rotation around the body axis, support and grasping functions of arms and hands, sitting up, kneeling, crawling, standing up, and walking. Examination of balancing reactions in all of these procedures of movement, including the intermediate steps. Observation of the quality of movements as well as of the amount of time needed to perform them. Examination of compensatory mechanisms.

● Examination of abnormal reactions to see whether abnormal tonic postural patterns exist and are influencing the child's motoricity.

● Examination of righting reactions.

● Examination of balancing reactions.

● Examination of skin sensitivity, skin color, and reaction to skin stimulation.

● Examination of perceptive ability of all senses as far as is possible by a physiotherapist, eventually consulting an occupational therapist or speech therapist.

● Examination of possible contractures and/or deformities.

● Examination of tone in all parts of the body. Recording of basic tone or changes of tone.

● Examination of the child's needs and psychological situation.

● Comprehension of the inner structure of the child's family through assessing the parents' needs as well as the expectations they place upon the child.

The Principles of Neurodevelopmental Therapy (Bobath)

Since the initially statically oriented treatment methods became more dynamic during the course of the past few years and this dynamism infiltrated the concept, one now speaks of "developmental treatment." From the term "reflex inhibiting initial position," the new term "reflex inhibiting pattern of movement" was coined by Bobath (1963).

The term "movement facilitation" blazed a trail. By inhibiting pathological, tonic postural patterns, tone is improved, and through facilitation of normal balancing reactions, a better feeling for movement is conveyed to the child. Inhibition and facilitation must be performed simultaneously.

Here, attention should be paid to so-called key points of movement, meaning head, shoulders, hips, and any proximally located joint with regard to the distal location. From these key points, sequences of movement can be controlled and influenced through stimulation. Using manipulating techniques which affect these key points, the extremities and, as a result, the entire child can move more freely and actively. This requires sensitive and well-developed empathy on the part of the therapist in order to take notice of and give consideration to the child's individual needs and capacity for free movement.

Among the additional treatment techniques are various methods of tapping:

- Inhibitory tapping

- Alternating tapping

- Stroke tapping

- Pressure tapping

Tapping techniques (light striking or knocking) spark impulses which, throught proprioceptive and tactile stimulation, influence the body's muscle tone. Here, summations of impulses are being dealt with which must be carried out in a certain sequence in order to produce the desired result. Should reflex patterns, associated reactions, or hypertonicity appear, the stimulation must be altered immediately. By combining reflex inhibition, facilitation, and/or stimulation and tapping, the attempt is made to direct central impulses into their correct tracks through feedback by way of peripheral stimuli.

It is important to realize that movement, whether it be more or less automatic or voluntary, is always carried out as rationally as possible, and each deviation demonstrates the difficulties with which the child is confronted. The method of treatment must always take this aspect into account.

According to Bobath (1963), the following are the objectives of treatment:

● Development of normal postural reactions and normal posture tone in order for the child to be able to hold itself in an upright position against the force of gravity and to control movements.

● To counteract the development of false reactions of posture and abnormal posture tone.

● To give the child a feeling for handling and play and to convey to it the functional patterns it will need to become independent in eating, washing, dressing, etc.

● Prevention of contractures and deformities.

The patterns of coordination, whose quality is decreased in children with motor disturbances, must be influenced as positively as possible through the treatment. Here, special emphasis is placed on the child's active movements.

The techniques of **facilitation** attempt to make the objective of these active automatic movements as easy as possible for the child to attain. The patterns of movement regarding motor development must be developed. This must take place passively—primarily through the therapist—by building up the patterns of movement to such an extent that the child can use them actively should it wish to do so. Early treatment gives us the opportunity of facilitating these patterns of movements so well that pathological patterns will not insert themselves. However, this depends on the extent of the damage. In this case, the therapist can reduce, develop, or maintain tone. Coordination of the antagonists or synergists can be regulated, and the nonfunctioning posture patterns can be slowed and facilitated into automatic or voluntary movements (facilis, Latin = easy, facilitate, make easier, pave the way for something).

Bobath (1961) summarizes the objectives of treatment as follows:

● It is necessary to have a normal postural reflex mechanism in order to achieve normal muscle tone for movement.

● This is constituted by the interaction of a large number of standing posture reflexes, particularly in the area of postural and equilibrium maintaining reflexes. These are subcortical, controlled processes, called "most automatic movements", meaning that these are movements which occur without the control of consciousness.

● Postural reflexes occur in the form of compensatory movements or changes in muscle tone which adapt to changes in posture, meaning that they do not necessarily initiate movements. In both cases, complex patterns of coordination are developed which originate above all from the least automatic, voluntary movements.

● These form the background which voluntarily executed movements require and with which sophisticated movements requiring motor function can be carried out. It builds up chronologically during the first 3 years of life. Postural reflexes are partially inhibited and partially replaced by the development of static reactions and voluntary actions, which are needed in the process of learning more sophisticated movements.

Despite all of the therapeutic techniques involving **inhibition and facilitation**, it is imperative to be certain that this handling leaves the child with the opportunity to move about actively on its own. Certainly, an inhibition should not lead to, for instance, the child no longer being able to move out of a given position. Here, facilitation at key points plays a major role so that the extent and distribution of insufficient and/or abnormal muscle tone can be controlled. This gives the child the possibility of moving from point to point. The therapist directs the key points of control. Thus, it may happen that inhibition and facilitation take place simultaneously. The therapist must observe this very precisely as the key points themselves cannot be actively moved by the child, but rather only from more distal points. This means that the therapist must continously adapt the program accordingly.

Due to the fact that the classic pattern of a motorically disturbed child who is still very young has not yet come to light, it is possible to prevent abnormal patterns of movement from inserting themselves by way of these techniques. These children learn to move about independently and do so using more normal patterns of movement from the very beginning.

At this point we re-emphasize the importance of observing the developmental sequence of flexion and extension and also the realization that it is sometimes possible to achieve the execution of functions from an extended, upright position which corresponds to earlier stages of development. Through the pressure and/or pull of gravity, the proprioceptors in the joints are sent the information for the upright position. Hence, a stabilization of tone, especially useful to a listless child for sequences of movement from the horizontal into the vertical position, occurs. Development of the intermediate stages of movement are therefore possible, which makes it easier for the children to react to normal stimuli and to adapt to their various degrees of difficulty.

This facilitation technique makes it possible for the child to carry out voluntary movements during the course of treatment without harsh intervention by the therapist. The therapist uses the key points to control the child's movements, thus allowing it to be active. Consequently, the child learns to control its positioning within a given space and is capable of reacting independently on all levels. Treatment may take place in any position; both the supine as well as the prone position are suitable, sitting, sitting sideways, kneeling, and standing. It should not be forgotten during treatment that extension is vital to attaining an upright position.

Treatment of children with motor disturbances is not complete until the sensorimotor system of perception has been included. Since sensomotoricity is constituted by the proprioceptive system of the muscles, tendons, and joints as well as the tactile-vestibular system itself, whereby one must differentiate between self and externally transmitted stimulation, treatment should be geared accordingly. Tactile and vestibular stimuli on all levels are techniques which can be very effectively utilized.

Additional Aids for Motor Therapy

Despite good physiotherapeutic treatment, there are some cases in which it is necessary to include a type of aid that will improve the success of treatment in combination with physiotherapy. The following describes those aids useful in early treatment but not of value for treating somewhat older children.

Lower-leg standing casts

Should danger of a contracture in the ankle joints exist, lower-leg standing casts are used, which are generally applied by an orthopedist. The child can walk about with it. A wooden plate is placed underneath the foot, which assures the foot's fixation upon the ground while stepping. The cast reaches only up to the lower limit of the knee joint and never covers more than one joint. The knee must remain free.

Application should be left to a specialist, because otherwise the feet could remain in a false position and become incorrigible. The toes should remain open. This type of treatment by cast must always be carried out on *both* legs so as not to encourage false perception.

Lower-leg standing cast treatment may not be commenced until skin sensitivity has been precisely diagnosed. Preparation for this type of cast therapy takes place during occupational therapy sessions, geared to whether hypersensitive or nonsensitive cutaneous sensibility in the legs and feet is present. The cast would feel uncomfortable or unbearable or even not be felt at all, which would decrease its therapeutic value or have an opposite effect. The success of therapy would thus not be assured.

Hammock

For children demonstrating an opisthotonic posture which appears to be surmountable, hammocks may sometimes prove themselves useful. Sometimes even an infant recliner, which is available in any department store, will suffice. If the child demonstrates competing tonic patterns of posture with extensive asymmetry, a hammock may cause damage. Using the trial-and-error method, one must try to place the child in the midline with a slight tilt. Swings and all sorts of objects in which a child can be moved convey to the child a feeling for its own system of balance (vestibular system) and may be used as long as they provide enjoyment. They also contribute to regulation of tone.

Positioning Vest (after Lübbe, 1976)

In rare cases, Lübbe's positioning vest can be used for scoliosis (determined in the sitting position). Here, as with a hammock, when competing tonic posture patterns are present, damage can be done. One must try it out in order to equalize a not yet fixed asymmetrical posture.

Hip Straddle/Expanding Apparatus

In cases of severe adductor spasm, one is tempted to work with expanding diapers, which can have disastrous effects. A hip-spreading pillow or Pavlik bandage are sometimes of help in such cases in order to prevent dislocation of the hip. Sometimes it is sufficient to dress the child in a double layer of diapers and to carry it on the hip. (Here, the mother should be sure to change the child's positioning from one hip to the other as otherwise the child assumes the mother's asymmetry; see "Directions for Handling.")

Thus, it becomes clear that the hip has a central function within the scope of this type of treatment. Extension and mobility of the hip—during the course of evolution and as a result of rising up against the force of gravity—have made the development of the brain and sight possible (and, subsequently, have made *Homo erectus* possible), which in turn has led to the development of modern man. This function of hip extension and mobility must be prepared very early, that is, before standing actually takes place, because this is necessary to achieve the upright position with simultaneous extension of the shoulder area.

This specific treatment must be included very early in movement facilitation. Otherwise, it is hardly possible to overcome flexion synergisms.

Here, the force of gravity through stimulation of the proprioceptors in the joints can help in attaining the stability needed for orderly motor function, particularly for intermediate steps of movement and with listless children.

"Handling" constitutes a significant component of the treatment as well. It aims to bring the child to react to influence from the environment with normal movements. This type of handling conveys to the child new sensory and motor experience of movement; subsequently, this affects the mother, who would otherwise support the child too intensively for too long a time, thus preventing it from gaining independence. The corresponding techniques, which the doctor can demonstrate to the mother, are described in the appendix to this book. A direkt correlation of this is specific training for the mother, or whomever the child relates to most closely in everyday routines, such as diaper changing, picking up, dressing, feeding, and bathing.

We are not concerned with merely showing the mother how to touch and move her child but, equally importantly, with simultaneously changing her into a kind of everready co-therapist by giving her detailed instructions regarding the method of treatment and pointing out her child's special psychological needs.

During the course of active treatment, one should pay attention to the fact that this constant manipulation can irritate the child considerably, if it is not given the chance to try out what it has experienced. This should occur continuously throughout treatment, particularly since, apart from motor improvement, sensory integration takes place. Learning processes do not occur purposelessly, but rather as Papoušek (1975) puts it, "learning toward success." The child is only able to obtain experience if it is permitted to try on its own. The well-known experience that a child may show improvement even after some weeks without treatment (e.g., vacation) should be taken as a guideline.

The therapist is dependent on "trial and error" and should learn to observe very precisely and always attempt to interpret correctly the phenomena arising. For the therapist this means a great amount of understanding for the changing situation of both the handicapped child and its family. In this respect, children with multiple handicaps represent a difficult problem. A physiotherapist capable of successfully treating such a child's motor handicaps frequently does not feel in a proper position—due to her/his specialized training and experience—to treat child's simultaneously existing sensory and proprioceptive disturbances with the same prospect of succeeding. For this reason, other therapists who are able to influence the associated deficiencies positively must be consulted so as not to place excessive demands on the one therapist.

On the other hand, experience has shown that during the first year of life a child should, if possible, be treated by only one person in order to avoid offering it too many "persons to relate to" other than the mother to whom the child must become accustomed.

According to the experience gained within the past few years, it can be concluded that occupational therapists, special educators, speech therapists, and other therapists are indeed capable of and successful in carrying out early treatment. Sometimes the different types of training the therapists have gone through, which they have practiced mainly on somewhat older children as opposed to infants, turn out to be unfavorable.

This requirement that single individuals offer comprehensive therapy to children with multiple handicaps can only be fulfilled if therapist training becomes more universal than has been the case. Therapists interested in this type of work, which is doubtless very satisfying, should be offered the opportunity of training as a "development therapist." Development therapist could be came a new profession. Building upon the foundation of his/her specific field of study, the therapist should have command of treatment techniques used by others in the field by way of a joint course of study. This therapist could become stimulated by the other areas of treatment while working with a child or be available to give advice, as he or she would become indispensible for the adequate treatment and training of a child whose handicaps have been diagnosed early.

We are dealing with a medical-psychological-pedagogical problem that requires imagination and commitment from all occupational groups belonging to this sector without singling out any one group to give it priority. All members of this "functional circle" are equal. It is this level of thought process that makes the indispensable "teamwork" possible. Also included in this circle are the parents and other persons constituting the child's environment, such as social workers, and who make therapy possible.

In a functional circle like this, the highly trained development therapist would represent the main figure. She/he would take up contact with all other members as necessary and coordinate their aid to the multiply handicapped child. She/he is also the one circle member to become visibly active on behalf of the child.

Normal and Deviating Development

First Month

Normal

Gross Motoricity

Supine position. While in the waking state (state 4), the flexion position prevails in small infants. The head tends to be slightly turned to the side; the body follows the turn en bloc. The arms are placed next to the body at a slight angle; the hands are partially open and partially closed in the prone position; the thumb is adducted, sometimes folded inwardly, yet always relaxed.

As long as flexion does not prevail, the shoulders lie somewhat retracted on the surface. The thorax is located in the midline and changes its position in accordance with the head position by way of the influence of the asymmetric tonic neck reaction (ATNR). Whenever the head moves, a Moro reaction may occur.

The legs lie outwardly rotated from the hips, sometimes only one leg, while the other may be laid on the side and even inwardly rotated. Either they are both abducted or they are both symmetrical, the one being abducted and the other adducted. The knees are bent, and the feet are dorsiflexed. Undifferentiated multiple movements still occur, overcoming the flexion pattern by way of the Moro reaction (Fig. **19**).

Fig. **19**

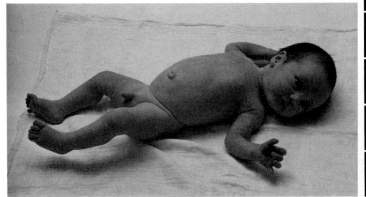

Prone position. In this placement, the flexion position also prevails. The knees lie underneath or nearly beside the trunk and are "freed" during extension out of the hip. The head usually lies to one side and can be briefly lifted to reposition it to the other side. Even without touching the child, preliminary crawling movements can be seen which appear alternately. Here, the trunk is moved in accordance with the head position.

The shoulders are either flexed or retracted slightly. The arms are either beneath or next to the thorax. The legs are outwardly rotated from the hips downward; the buttocks are slightly lifted. The knees are flexed, and the feet are dorsiflexed (Fig. **20**).

Fig. **20**

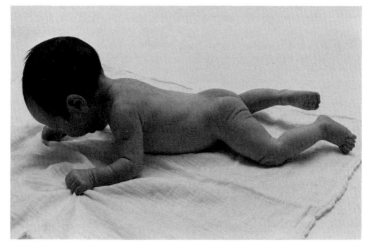

Pulling up from the supine position. If the child is slowly pulled upward and forward, the arms remain flexed, and the head hangs toward the back. As soon as the vertical, supported sitting position is attained, the head falls forward and totters from one side to the other (Figs. **21**, **22**).

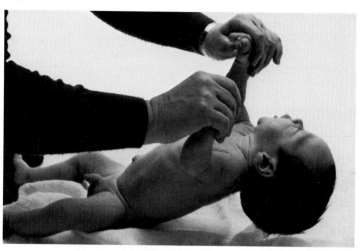

Fig. **21**

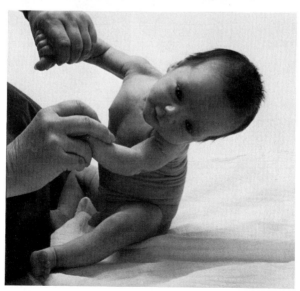

Fig. **22**

Setting the child on its feet while giving support under the armpits. The child seems to put its weight down—however, this cannot be ascertained—and then collapses with flexed knees (physiological astasia) (Figs. **23, 24**).

Fig. **23**   Fig. **24**

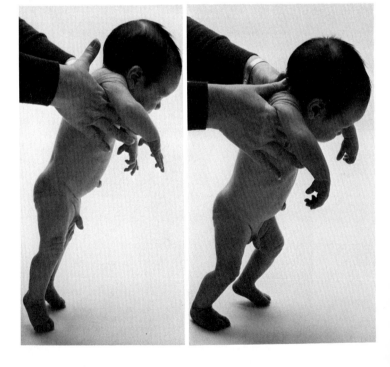

1

Posture and Muscle Tone

When merely looking at the child without touching it, the flexion tone prevails and is not easy to overcome, even when the child is only passively moved. Distinct resistance to extension exists. The extended extremities return to the initial position when they are released.

Placing Reactions

There is only limited ability of adjusting head placement. The child does not yet adapt to each change of position. Its posture is primarily determined by gravity.

Balancing Reactions

In testing the horizontal and vertical positions, no balance can as yet be ascertained. Every reaction the child demonstrates while being moved through a room should be observed as well as whether the baby enjoys these movements or cries. Observe both the intensity of and the threshold at which the Moro reaction appears.

Symmetry

The child is in a nearly symmetrical lying position with slight turning of the head towards its "favorite" side. As the child takes up this position, there is still an influence of the position in utero and during birth.

Tonic Patterns of Posture, Reflexes, and Reactions of Early Infancy

The influence of posture patterns are sometimes visible at this age. During passive examining of turning the head to one side, the extremities on the facial side sometimes extend while the extremities of the occipital side flex. At times this is more readily visible in the legs than in the arms.

All reflexes and reactions previously described can be triggered off with equal ease on both sides as long as the examining conditions are kept constant.

Fine Motor Function and Adaptation

Moving objects in the line of visibility (not too close, the distance should be about 40–50 cm) are perceived and focused on, although for only a very short time. The child's eyes and head will follow an object after stimulation through another object or the mother's face to the midline, but not further.

The child reacts to bright light or loud noise by frowning, crying, or a Moro reaction or lessens its activities and becomes completely tranquil.

Speech and Social Contact

Speech. An infant can produce a few involuntary laryngeal sounds as well as snorkling noises at night. It cries before meals but is immediately pacified when feeding begins. If a bell is rung, the infant becomes quiet and attentive.

Social contact. During the first month, the child has an almost immobile face (amimia) with a smile "sparking up" every now and then for no apparent reason. Sometimes it looks at its mother or the examiner. Noises quickly startle it. Motor activity and multiple movements are prevented when the child is distracted. The child is pacified by being picked up or caressed, when it hears a familiar voice, by body warmth, and when being nursed, causing it to open its mouth.

Hearing and Localizing Sounds

When the child hears noises, it interrupts its movements; however, it does not immediately turn towards the location from whence the noise comes. Sometimes the child begins to cry after the noise ceases.

Sound Formation with Special Attention Given to Breathing, Sucking, and Swallowing

The infant can produce involuntary laryngeal sounds. It cries loudly when it feels hunger or becomes tired; it has a forceful voice. Breathing is regular. Sucking and swallowing are well coordinated.

Visison and Eye Movements

The infant takes notice of objects that move if they remain at a distance of 40–50 cm, and it focuses on them briefly. Eye movement is not yet well coordinated; occasional strabismus appears (crossed eyes).

Emotional Behavior

If the examination conditions are optimal, the child should be basically peaceful, awake, and attentive. Its eyes are open, and occasionally it smiles. At this age the parents' anxieties during the examination play an important role in the child's behavior. Should the child cry, one should be capable of putting oneself in the parent's place and of giving them suitable advice as the parents are frequently anxious in the presence of a doctor. The child is usually pacified by the mother's voice and the warmth she radiates.

Deviating Development

Gross Motoricity

Supine position. Either the child's normally flexed posture is too evident, or the child already demonstrates a too distinct extension at this age. These patterns can be complete, or they may show preferences such as over extension at the shoulders, legs, or hips. In the case of extensive flexion, every movement to attain another position takes place en bloc; in the case of extension, rotation is made exceedingly difficult. The shoulders should be observed as they may be overly retracted. The child's arms may take up extreme positions and demonstrate asymmetrical patterns. There may be exaggerated inward or outward shoulder rotation. The arms often rest in a pronated position. On the whole, there are unmodifiable, complete patterns of movement.

The child's hands are closed to form a fist. The thumb is usually tucked in and adducted at the basal joint. A strongly extended trunk with asymmetrical posture should be considered a deviation. In these cases, the legs are inwardly rotated and adducted. They cannot escape from this position. All movements are reduced and sometimes even impossible. The child lies very quietly. If the child is extremely limp, its body rests completely upon the surface of the pad. Whenever the child wishes to move itself, it does so with much effort.

The movements are exaggerated, restless gestures. The legs lie in the frog position with a strong outward rotation from the hips. Overextension should most likely be seen as an attempt by the child to move itself; however, the extent to which this actually is such an attempt cannot be exactly ascertained. The movement, therefore, turns out to be too extreme and demonstrates too much extension (Fig. **25**).

Fig. **25**

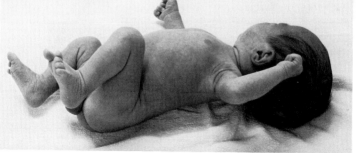

Prone position. Flexion posture may appear to such a great extent when in the prone position that the child may no longer be capable of lifting its head. This would make the development of extension impossible as this is normally initiated by the head. During the course of further development, the child does not come to support its weight on its lower arms, since the pull of gravity cannot be overcome. The child cannot turn its head to the side freely, which results in incomplete functioning of the respiratory system, and the child has difficulty breathing. The child does not learn to adjust its head and body within space; the ability to do so at this age is necessary for future development.

Through this complete pattern, alternating movements that are considered a kind of "preparatory program" for alternating locomotion are not possible. The immobility of the legs—whether due to hyper- or hypotonia—has the effect of preventing the child from discovering its legs and feet as a part of its body and thus from using them meaningfully (Fig. **26**).

Fig. **26**

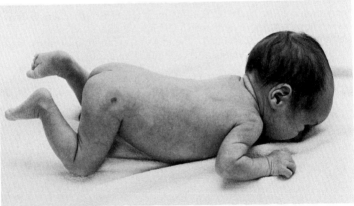

Pulling up from the supine position. It is by no means easy to grasp the palms of the child's hands, because either the hand is so tightly closed that one is unable to get a finger inside or the examiner's finger slips out as the child does not grasp it. The grasping reaction must be overcome—a feat that can prove to be quite difficult. When pulling the child up forward, the child's arms are either flexed to such a great extent that it can be pulled up completely without any effort on the child's part or the arms are completely extended since hypotonia does not allow flexion.

Although an infant of this age does not yet possess head control, it still becomes obvious in cases where deviations are present that even the limited amount of tone that is usually present is lacking, making the head fall listlessly in all directions (Fig. 27).

At times the head seems "trapped" between the shoulders, and the shoulder area is blocked.

Fig. **27**

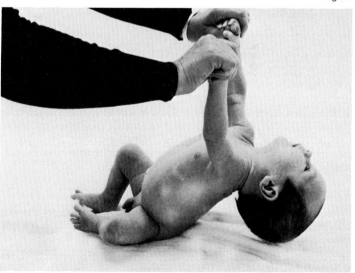

Setting the child on its feet while giving support under the armpits. The child's legs are stretched either too strongly or insufficiently toward the underlying surface (Fig. **28**).

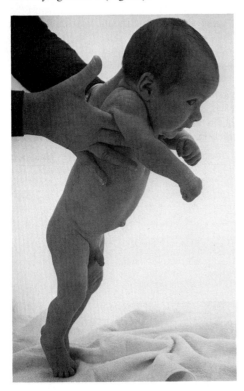

Fig. **28**

Reflexes and reactions. All reflexes and reactions appear too active or do not appear at all even if optimal examining conditions are maintained. Reactions are asymmetrical (when observing physiological asymmetries). The infant reacts either with apathy or with overexcitability when an attempt is made to induce reflexes.

Fine Motor Function and Adaptation

When dealing with deviations from the norm, one can observe that the child does not perceive items clearly enough. At times one has the impression that the child is blind or deaf as the stimuli go through no centralized processing. The child's reactions to light and noise are either exaggerated or inadequately low.

1

Speech and Social Contact

Speech. It is sometimes noticed that the infant is either too passive or too restless. It either cries incessantly or not at all. The former worries the members of the child's environment more than the latter, hence stimulating more attention.

Social contact. At this age, it is sometimes not noticed that the infant does not take up enough contact with its environment. In such cases, the mother's comments should be carefully noted as she has a feeling for the difficulties the child has in establishing contact with its environment. Of course, the difficulty may be due to a hearing or vision disturbance. It sometimes happens that the child does not react adequately to attempts to pacify it through caressing, by picking it up, through warmth or nursing.

Posture and Muscle Tone

The quality of the tone is distinctly noticeable in a child's posture and during examination. The child demonstrates either too much flexion or too much extension. Furthermore, it may lie listlessly and move either too much or too little. Asymmetries can be observed well in the child's posture. When double-checking, one notices differences in tone.

Righting Reactions

Although at this age righting reactions are still poor, a child demonstrates extreme situations if a deviation is present. Even the little amount of reactivity that is necessary to overcome gravity cannot or can hardly be carried out by a child with conspicuous signs.

Balancing Reactions

Since a child does not yet have balance at that age, deviations cannot be recognized. Every reaction the child demonstrates when it is moved within space should be observed as well as whether the child is enjoying itself or crying. The intensity and threshold of the triggering of a Moro reaction should be noted.

Symmetry

The most striking factor of all regarding recognition of abnormality of motor development at this age seems to be symmetry. Very distinct asymmetries should be recognized as a hemisyndrome and call for exact observation. One should carry out an intensive search for the causes at this age as sometimes it is merely a clinical indication of the basic illness. One must bear in mind, though, that malpositioning in utero or during birth can be the cause of asymmetries.

Tonic Patterns of Posture, Reflexes, and Reactions of Early Infancy

In the case of abnormalities, the influences of tonic patterns of posture are no longer the issue at hand, but persisting reactions are. They always remain constant and are very intensive and can often be triggered off asymmetrically. When triggering reflexes and reactions, it should be observed whether or not they are asymmetrical and what degree of intensity they have—either too strong or too weak. In cases of apathy or hyperexcitability syndrome as well as in hypotonia, hypertonia, and hemisyndromes, these reflexes and reactions are always conspicuous (Fig. **29**).

Fig. **29**

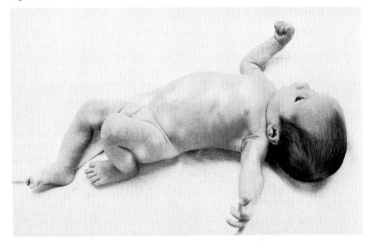

Emotional Behavior

Even when constant examining conditions are maintained, deviations are recognizable in a child's behavior. These children become either exceedingly quiet or restless. A child's smile is a good indicator and should be continuously observed.

It is sometimes impossible to either pacify or activate such a child.

Hearing and Localizing Sounds

Not only hearing defects can be the cause of a lack of reaction in a child, disturbances in centralized processing may also be the reason.

Sound Formation with Special Attention Given to Breathing, Sucking, and Swallowing

Observe whether or not the child "forms" any sounds. A spastic disturbance of coordination can be the reason for a lack of sound formation. A listless child may also lack sound formation. Crying is either very shrill or quietly forced. Poor, irregular breathing and faulty coordination during sucking or swallowing are signs of a severe handicap.

Vision and Eye Movements

Deficiencies in processing are possible not only through disturbances in visual function but also on a centralized level, which means that vision and fixation in any area must be observed well. Eye coordination, which has not yet achieved full function at this age, is often more disturbed in children with abnormalities (fluctuating strabismus).

Second Month

Normal

Gross Motoricity

Supine position. The child still demonstrates flexion posture; however, extension has improved. It kicks alternately, and only seldomly both legs at the same time. It turns its head to one side (mostly to its favorite side), but the head can be turned to the other side. The arms are at an angle next to the body; the hands are open. Sometimes the arms are raised but not yet to such an extent that they reach the midline.

The body lies symmetrically, and sometimes retractions on the side of the trunk toward which the face is turned can be noted. The legs are outwardly rotated from the hips and are sometimes well abducted. They can be placed together on both sides; one side is frequently more inwardly rotated than the other. Mass movements have subsided; a Moro reaction is still sometimes triggered off by head movements (Fig. 30) as an expression of vestibular stimulation.

Fig. **30**

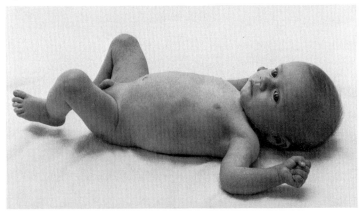

Prone position. At 2 months of age, flexor tone still prevails, but the child is able to extend in the thorax area. The hip is still bent. The child lifts its head—still a bit shakily—for a short moment, but not yet more than 45°.

The shoulders are still somewhat retracted. The arms are bent—not yet in a stable manner—with the lower arms, which serve as support, on the ground. The buttocks are slightly lifted as a result of hip flexion and the physiological flexion tendency. The legs are outwardly rotated from the hips on and kick alternately; the feet are mostly dorsiflexed but can also be plantarflexed (Fig. **31**).

Fig. **31**

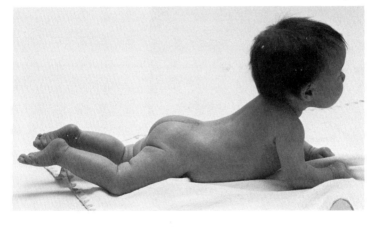

Pulling the child up from the supine position. When the child is taken by the hands and slowly pulled up and forward, its arms flex slightly. The child is already quite good at pulling the head up and forward with its body. When the upright sitting position is reached, the child's head falls slightly forward and is shakily directed into the more stable, upright position. The trunk is still somewhat unstable but symmetrical. A slight amount of postural asymmetry depends on tone and ATNR (physiological) (Fig. 32–34).

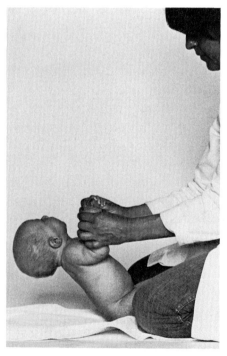

Fig. **32**

2

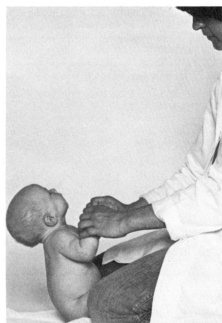

Fig. **33**

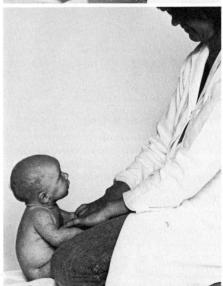

Fig. **34**

Setting the child on its feet while giving support under the armpits. The child holds its body weight for only a short time but has become more stable. It easily collapses with flexed knees (Fig. **35**).

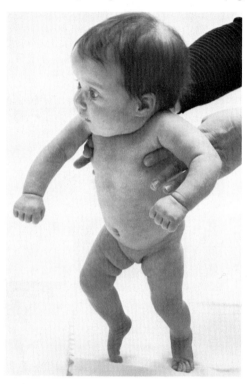

Fig. **35**

Posture and Muscle Tone

The flexion tone has decreased. It is easily overcome during passive examination. When extension occurs against flexion, there is no longer great resistance; however, the extended extremity swings back into the original position after it has been set free.

Righting Reactions

The child is already able to adjust its head within space quite nicely in all positions, although its head is still a bit shaky. When in a prone position, the child lifts its head by way of the labyrinthine righting reaction. The influence of gravity which the child must combat loses some of its effect; the child is already capable of adapting to changes in its position within space for a short period.

Balancing Reactions

The child becomes more stable in both the supine and prone position; its balancing reactions improve. If the child loses its balance, it tries to adapt to the new situation; however, it is not yet successful enough at this. It is a pleasure to the child to be moved about—the child smiles or seems to feel pleased. Being moved about through the environment has either a stimulating or pacifying effect.

2

Symmetry

The child can lie symmetrically and move itself. A certain amount of physiological asymmetry due to brain dominance and dependent upon tonus in posture and tonic patterns of posture (favorite side) can become visible.

Tonic Patterns of Posture and Reactions of Early Infancy

The influence of tonic patterns of posture, such as ATNR, TLR, and STNR are also visible at this age. However, they do not interfere with the coordination of movements. Reactions are less intense but easily triggered off on both sides.

Fine Motor Function and Adaptation

Moving objects in the line of vision (at a distance of 30–40 cm) are taken notice of and focused upon. The eyes remain fixed on the object until it leaves the line of vision. The child's eyes follow a stimulus, usually accompanied by a head movement. The child's glance reaches the midline and, for a short period, passes it.

The child reacts to irritation by extremely bright light by frowning and wrinkling its forehead, through a Moro reaction, or by decreasing its activity. The child then becomes very quiet.

Grasping

The child's hands are usually formed into a loosely closed fist. Frequently, the child puts its whole hand or just its thumb into its mouth. The child's hand opens when touched, for instance, by a rattle. The rattle is then held tightly but not yet let go of (palmar grasping reflex).

Speech and Social Contact

Speech. The infant can produce several sounds (a, e, o, u). Sometimes these sounds are connected by using an "h" (ha, he, ehe). The infant's laugh may turn into borborygmus. The infant reacts to smiling by changing its facial expression. Crying becomes more differentiated and denotes moods. If a bell rings, the infant turns toward the noise. The child remains peaceful and becomes attentive.

Social contact. The child already takes up contact with its environment when it is spoken to. It smiles and attentively observes faces that do not come too close. The child is dependent upon its environment for producing reactions, and it indeed reacts to, for instance, pacifying if it is picked up or hears a familiar voice.

Hearing and Localizing Sounds

Whenever the child hears noises, it ceases its movements. It may also turn toward the origin of the noise. Sometimes it begins to cry when the noise ceases.

Sound Formation with Special Attention Given to Breathing, Sucking, and Swallowing

Infants already form several sounds such as long and short "a, o, u." At times these vowels are connected together by an "h." Laughing may convert to borborygmus; the infant screeches. The infant cries loudly whenever it is hungry and whimpers to itself whenever it is tired. The child's whimpering can have various expressions. Depending upon the reason, it cries with a loud or with a soft voice. The voice is powerful, and breathing is regular. Sucking and swallowing are well coordinated.

Vision and Eye Movements

The infant takes note of objects that move about in front of it at a distance of 30–40 cm and focuses upon them for a short period of time. The eye movements approach the midline and even briefly cross it. Eye movements are not yet fully coordinated; only rarely does strabismus occur.

Emotional Behavior

If conditions for examination can be kept constant, the child should be basically peaceful, wide-eyed, and attentive. Its eyes are open; from time to time the child smiles. The parents' anxieties play an important role in the child's behavior. A calming consultation with the parents often has the same effect upon the infant.

Deviating Development

Gross Motoricity

Supine position. The flexion posture, which is still physiological, is stronger, or the child does not show the amount of extension normal at this age. These patterns are most striking when they are total. Preference of sectors such as, for instance, the shoulder area or the hips and legs is common. Movements from the flexed position occur en bloc. In the case of an extension pattern, rotation is either not possible at all or only barely existent. No alternating kicking can be observed. The head is held asymmetrically; sometimes extensive flexion toward one side is preferred, sometimes additional extension is present, which is called the opisthotonic posture.

The shoulders are strongly retracted, and the hands are balled to a fist. The arms are held in extremely asymmetrical poses—either too strongly bent or too strongly extended. The arms and hands take on an emphatic prone position. Patterns of movement are not modifiable and hence are always total. The infant's closed hands have adducted, turned-in thumbs.

Extensive extension of the trunk with an asymmetrical posture should be considered abnormal.

The legs are frequently inwardly rotated from the hips and adducted. This position is often fixed and cannot be overcome by the child alone.

If the child is extremely floppy, its entire body will touch the surface of the pad. If the child does move, the movements appear overmodulated, meaning that they seem very disquieted and jolting. The legs are in a frog position as far as the hips, demonstrate excessive outward rotation, and are abducted.

Overextension should most likely be considered an attempt to move about, without the ability to estimate the degree of movement; hence, the movement becomes extreme and therefore demonstrates excessive extension (Fig. **36**).

Fig. **36**

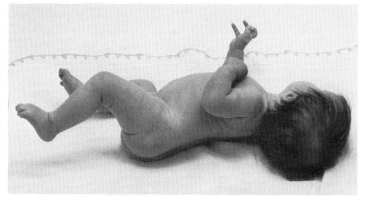

Prone position. In the prone position flexion may be so great that the child has difficulties in or is completely prevented from lifting its head. In this case the development of extension, which is initiated by the head, is no longer possible.

Support by leaning on the lower arms is either difficult or impossible. The child does not move its head to the side enough or, in some cases, not at all, so the respiratory system becomes obstructed. The child's head positioning in space is awkward, which leads to difficulties in the development of a body image as well as of the child's positioning of itself in space.

Figs. **37, 38**

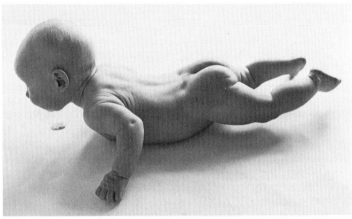

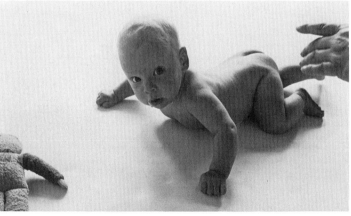

Due to the total pattern, alternating movements—a kind of "prepro-gram" for walking—are not possible. The immobility of the child's legs—whether due to hypotonia or hypertonia—prevents the child from discovering its legs as a part of its body. The same holds true for the child's feet (Figs. **37, 38**).

Pulling upward from the supine position. Due to the firmly closed hands or the limp tone, it is very difficult for the examiner to take up contact with the palms of the child's hands in order to stimulate it into helping pull itself upward. Sometimes the child demonstrates a grasp-ing reflex that is still too strong. While pulling the child up and for-ward, its arms are either flexed to such a great degree that the child can be pulled up with no effort at all on its part or its arms are stretched in complete listlessness since hypotonus prevents flexion.

Although an infant at this age does not necessarily possess head con-trol, it nevertheless becomes obvious in deviating cases that even the smallest amount of tonicity is missing, and the child's head hangs limply in all directions (Fig. **39**). Sometimes the child's head seems "walled in," and the shoulder area demonstrates blockage.

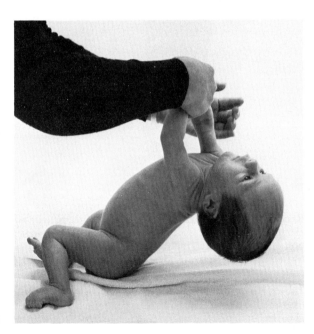

Fig. **39**

Setting the child on its feet while giving support under its armpits: The child either stretches its legs too extensively (positive supporting reaction) or too little (astasia) toward the pad (Fig. **40**).

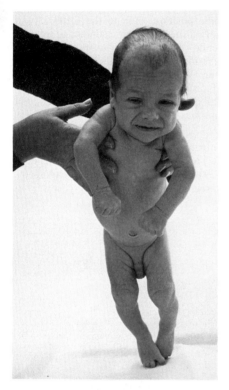

Fig. **40**

Reactions: All reactions appear either too excessive or not at all. The examiner should take care to find out whether physiological degeneration or even an early kind of suppression of such reactions is present. Most important is to insure that examining conditions be arranged optimally.

The reactions appear quite asymmetrical (not the physiological asymmetries of this age). The child reacts either by demonstrating apathy or hyperexcitability when an attempt is made to trigger the reactions.

Fine Motor Function and Adaptation

In cases of deviation from the norm, one can observe that the child does not perceive objects to the extent it should. At times it even seems as if the child were deaf or blind since the stimuli are not adequately processed by the central nervous system.

The child's reactions to light and noise are either exaggerated or inadequate.

As a result of shoulder retraction, the child is unable to make its hands meet at the midline.

Speech and Social Contact

Speech. The child utters only a few or no sounds at all. It does not laugh and squeal as is normal at this age, even in response to stimulation (do not get too close to the child; a minimum distance of 30–40 cm must be kept).

The infant cries in a shrill voice or not at all, or only whines quietly. No differentiation of crying occurs. It does not turn if a bell is rung. The child cries incessantly which makes the people in its environment become uneasy and results in the child becoming all the more timid.

Social contact. The child does not take up contact with its environment. There is no reaction to smiles if it is approached, and no observance of its surroundings.

Posture and Muscle Tone

The child's tone is conspicuous in posture as well as in any examining situation. Excessive flexion or extension can be observed sometimes to different degrees at the top or bottom part of the body. The child may just lie listlessly on the pad and move about too much or too little. When the attempt is made to extend the arms, one observes that this is either only possible with great difficulty or the arm quickly returns to the initial position. There is a kind of asymmetry in posture that can be felt as a difference in tone during examination.

Righting Reactions

There is a lack of positioning of the head or the body in space. Sometimes it is faintly perceptible, but not to a sufficient extent. The child is still very much subject to the influence of gravity, making attainment of an upright position seem difficult. For this reason, the child is not readily capable of adapting to a change of its position in space.

Balancing Reactions

As of yet, there are no indications pointing toward a stabilization in the supine and prone positions and no reestablishment of balance after having lost it. All reactions the infant makes while being moved about in space should be observed, and it should also be noted whether the child seems to enjoy the movement or whether it cries. Observe both the intensity and threshold of the Moro reaction.

All movement is pleasant for the infant. The child smiles all the while and appears to be enjoying itself. Being moved about in its surroundings has either a calming or a stimulating effect upon the child.

Symmetry

The infant is not capable of taking up a symmetrical position; one side is always preferred and the child is not able to change this by itself (always keep in mind the physiological asymmetry of this age).

Tonic Patterns of Posture and Reactions of Early Infancy

Tonic patterns of posture persist to an intractably strong degree, thereby preventing coordination of movement. Strong ATNR, at times asymmetrical TLR, and STNR are present, which cannot be triggered off at all or only excessively and do not occur symmetrically (Fig. **41**).

Fig. **41**

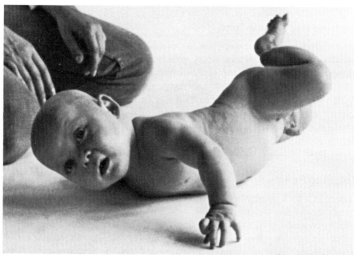

Emotional Behavior

The child cries frequently and piercingly during the examination. It is timid and cannot be calmed. It does not smile when addressed by another person. Even after the parents have been calmed, the child remains uneasy.

2

Hearing and Localizing Sounds

One does not receive the impression that the child hears or localizes noises. Sometimes only one side reacts, while the other does nothing. This may be due to a disturbance in centralized processing.

Sound Formation with Special Attention Given to Breathing, Sucking, and Swallowing

There is a complete lack of or inadequate sound formation, including little borborygmus or squealing. The child's crying does not demonstrate distinct differentiation. When crying, the child's voice is sometimes pathetically whining or piercing.

Breathing is irregular and poor, and coordination of sucking and swallowing is not good. The child's mouth is often open and obviously slobbering. The tongue is very stiff in the case of hypertonicity. In the case of hypotonicity, the lower lip hangs down.

Vision and Eye Movements

No perception of objects or persons is obvious. This can be due not only to blindness but also to a deficiency in centralized processing. During the examination, the child does not move its eyes beyond the midline. Substantial strabismus persists.

Grasping

The child's hands are consistently balled into a fist and open only very sluggishly and with poor extension in the fingers. The child does not suck either its fingers or its entire hand. A rattle that touches the child's hand is not grasped, or, if it is, it takes a great effort to get it out of the child's hold (grasping reflex is too strong).

Third Month

Normal

Gross Motoricity

Supine position. The infant can lie symmetrically on its back and move itself to both sides. Turning no longer occurs en bloc but rather with a certain amount of rotation. The head can be held in mid-position; however, the child frequently prefers to lie with its head on one particular side, and in doing so, the trunk is contracted on the side toward which the face is directed, causing an asymmetrical position to be assumed. It can be overcome, though. Here, the influences of the ATNR (Fig. **42**) are evident. The hands can be moved to the mid-line and looked at. The fingers are open, and they close whenever the bent arms are laid next to the body and the shoulders retracted.

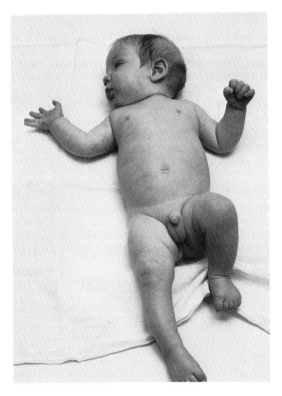

Fig. **42**

The child plays with its hands and is able to hold a rattle that is placed into its hand. It tries to put the rattle into its mouth. The child does not yet let go of the rattle, but rather occasionally it coincidently lets the rattle fall if the hands open as they do during the Moro reaction.

The child's legs are outwardly rotated from the hips in abduction with flexion. Alternate kicking is possible. At times, the knees are extended, and the child's feet are very mobile at the ankle joint.

Mass movements have become somewhat sparser, and all movements seem more coordinated. The child sometimes already lies in an extended position, but the position changes constantly.

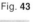

When the child performs active movements with its head, a Moro reaction may sometimes occur with abduction and outward rotation of the arms during which the hands open.

Prone position. The child lies symmetrically on the surface and is capable of spontaneously changing from an asymmetrical to a symmetrical position. It lifts its head up to 45°. Support through the lower arms is not yet stable. The head can be laid from one side to the other and can be moved. Sometimes the child falls over in doing so. The child's hands are balled into fists which can be opened; however, this seems usually to occur involuntarily. Incipient extension in the area of the neck and thorax is present. The hips are better extended but still often flexed, and as a result, the buttocks are frequently raised. The child kicks alternatingly along the trunk axis. The legs are outwardly rotated and abducted, the feet are dorsiflexed or extended, and the ankle joint is mobile. The knees are flexed (Fig. **43**).

Fig. **43**

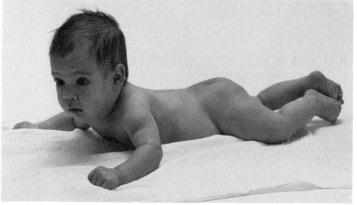

Pulling up from the supine position. The child helps when being pulled up even though its head control is not yet quite stable. The head accompanies the body when being pulled quite well but still totters slightly to and from. However, in the upright position, the child's head no longer falls forward, backward or to the side in an uncontrolled manner. The head is held at mid-position to the trunk. The legs follow forward but are still flexed at the knees.

In the upright position, the trunk is more stable, but the back is not yet fully extended. The child's arms are bent at the elbow when the child is being pulled up and forward and one can feel the child's tug. No extension for support takes place yet. If the child is held at the waist and tilted somewhat to one side, the child's head is already capable of repositioning itself horizontally in space quite nicely, despite the fact that it is sometimes quite slow and not really symmetrical, depending upon which is its favorite side (Figs. **44–46**).

Fig. **44**

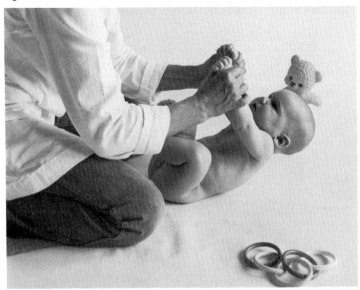

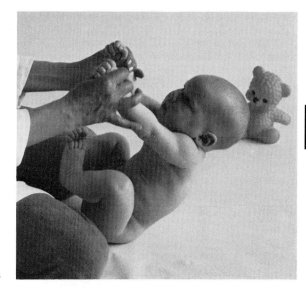

Fig. **45**

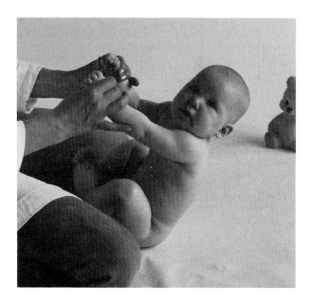

Fig. **46**

Setting the child on its feet while giving support under its armpits. The child is able to put its weight on its feet and legs for a short period. The child has also become more stable in standing. Its legs demonstrate contraction, the knees are straightened, and there is hip movement. The trunk is extended, and the child's head is better controlled and positions itself well in space (Fig. **47**).

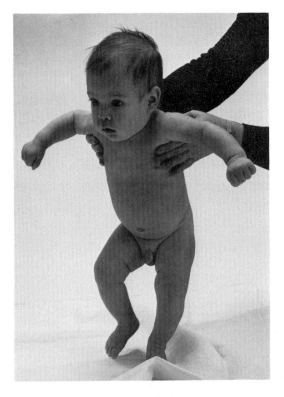

Fig. **47**

Posture and Muscle Tone

Flexion tone no longer prevails; the child starts to demonstrate patterns of extension. In passive examination, normal tone is seen which is sometimes slightly looser and sometimes slightly firmer, but there is good mobility and no limitations. Passively extended extremities no longer swing back into the initial position; instead, they remain in the position they were placed in.

Shoulder and hip tension should be examined as well as flexibility in the trunk toward each side in both the supine and prone positions. Test for resistance against extension.

Righting Reactions

The child is already able to adjust its head quite well in all positions (this test should be carried out in the prone position, in the supine position, with sideways repositioning, and in the hanging position). The child is not yet capable of adapting to a change of its position in space over a long period of time; however, this capacity has improved decisively.

Balancing Reactions

The child is more stable in all positions; test first in the supine position, then in the prone position, and finally in the upright position. When the child loses its balance, it does attempt to adapt; however, the attempts are not yet successful enough. No support reaction takes place, but there is an initial extending of the arms toward the pad with clenched fists and flexed elbow joints. No transfer of body weight can be noted. Any reaction the child shows while being moved about in space should be observed as well as whether the child seems to enjoy the movements or whether it cries. The intensity of and threshold at which the Moro reaction is triggered off should be observed as well.

Any type of movement is perceived by the child as a pleasurable experience; the child usually smiles or just appears delighted. Being moved about in its surroundings has either a stimulating or pacifying effect upon the child.

Symmetry

The child is capable of resting in any position with a certain amount of symmetry; nonetheless, in a physiological sense it sometimes rests in an asymmetrical position. From this position, however, it can change to a different one; there are no limitations of coordination of movement. If the child is set down while being held, sometimes a slight type of surmountable scoliosis posture may be noticeable. This holds especially true when dealing with a somewhat slack child.

The child frequently has a "favorite side," which is usually the right.

Tonic Patterns of Posture and Reactions in Early Infancy

Influences of tonic patterns of posture, such as ATNR, TLR, and rarely STNR, are frequently still distinctly visible at this age. However, they do not hamper the coordination of movements. Reflexes and primary reactions either cannot be triggered at all or only very rarely. Hardly any palmar grasping reflex remains; the plantar reflex is still easily triggered.

The Moro reaction may still be present, even if only the first phase. At times, only the hands are open. The righting reaction can still be triggered, and there is no stepping reaction. (In prematurely born children, reflexes and reactions can still be triggered without any pathological significance even considering the gestational age.)

Fine Motor Function and Adaptation

Objects are taken notice of at the midline and beyond on both sides within the field of vision at a distance of 30–40 cm. The child follows an object through an angle of 180°. The child no longer only glances at the object briefly, but rather takes an interest in it (e.g., by interrupting its movement). The eyes are kept on the object. Eye and head movement are frequently coordinated simultaneously.

If the child's hands are touched, they open and grasp for the rattle being presented. The rattle is then moved about and let go of by accident.

The child looks at its hands and lifts them over its head with bent arms. The child takes its thumb or a single finger into its mouth, but no longer the entire hand.

Grasping

The child is able to grasp a rattle that is presented to it in a rather uncoordinated manner. Substantial pronation and palmar, total grasp are still evident. The rattle is held and moved about. The child looks at the rattle and repeats the movement. Then the child's hand falls down by accident, while not yet letting go. The child can join its hands together at the midline.

Speech and Social Contact

Speech. The child laughs loudly whenever it is spoken to. It turns its head toward the person speaking and gurgles and squeals spontaneously. It is delighted about the sounds it makes. It produces blow-friction noises by pressing air through its closed lips. The noise resembles an f, w, s, or th.

The child's crying is differentiated and indicates moods. The child turns toward a noise and becomes very quiet and attentive.

Social contact. The child looks at the examiner quite firmly and smiles when given words of encouragement. It follows people with its eyes. It observes the faces turned toward it very precisely. The child is dependent upon the reactions of its environment; for instance, it perceives an anxious mother or a hectic pace in the surroundings and reacts accordingly. If it cries, it allows itself to be pacified by being picked up, by being caressed, and through body warmth.

3

Hearing and Localizing Sounds

When the child hears noises, it stops whatever it is doing, and sometimes it even turns toward the source of the sound. The noises used in testing should be of various qualities, such as a bell, a soft voice, rustling paper, a bleep sound, music, etc. If the noise is very loud, the child sometimes cries when the noise ceases.

Sound Formation with Special Attention Given to Breathing, Sucking, and Swallowing

The infant forms additional sounds that are similar to an f, w, s, or th. It makes blow-friction noises by pressing air through its closed lips. It laughs and squeals and is delighted at the noises it produces and repeats them. The child cries loudly and with a husky voice when it is hungry or tired. Breathing is regular, and sucking and swallowing are well coordinated. The child's crying is of varying expression depending upon the cause (intense or whining).

Vision and Eye Movements

The infant looks at objects at a distance of 30–40 cm and follows them through an angle of 180° with both its eyes and by turning its head. Eye movements are coordinated; very rarely is strabismus noted.

Emotional Behavior

The child should preferably be in state 4; any deviations must be clearly documented. The child smiles at the examiner whenever it is not afraid of a stranger. As early as at this age, such reactions can appear. Nevertheless, the child allows itself to be calmed down quite quickly by being picked up or caressed, hearing a soft voice, and feeling body warmth. For this reason, the examination may begin on the mother's lap.

Development

Although not yet to a sufficient degree, a much more stable type of behavior has developed out of the formerly very unstable behavior. A modified pattern with extension has arisen from the previous total flexion, but flexion still prevails.

Positioning of the head in space improves, especially when the child is in an upright position. The child considers its new found capabilities pleasant and signals this to its environment.

Thus, mental development becomes possible, which can be clearly observed by looking at the child's lively eyes. Motor capacity is still insufficient. The child would like to explore more of its environment than it is capable of doing from a motor point of view. The people that make up its environment are called upon to fill this gap. Social behavior is developed in this way, particularly towards the parents. The child wants to be addressed and held.

Deviating Development

Gross Motoricity

Supine position. The child often lies in an asymmetrical position, and through this as well as overextended flexion patterns, it is often only able to turn to one side or not able to turn at all. The child cannot hold its head in the midline sufficiently. ATNR and TLR often appear jointly, which leads to patterns of posture that completely prevent any type of coordination of movement. Distinct shoulder retraction along with fisted hands prevents the child from joining its hands above its chest which, in turn, negates the development of hand-eye coordination.

If objects are put into the mouth, it is only with great effort. The Moro reaction may occur so intensively that it prevents all grasping function as anything the child may have in its hands falls out again.

The child's legs are either inwardly rotated and adducted or in a frog position. Sometimes they take up a very primitive position, merely bent at the knees but with no alternating kicking movement.

Extensor or flexor posture is seen in the nearly immobile ankles. The child rarely changes its position, since with hypertonia or hypotonia it cannot overcome gravity. In cases of hypertonia, extensive flexor or extensor tone can appear (Fig. **48**).

Fig. **48**

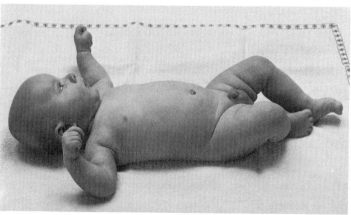

Prone position. In the prone position as well, slight or severe incorrect postures form extreme patterns. The posture is frequently asymmetrical. The child either hardly lifts its head at all or far too much.

Supporting itself upon the lower arms—a feat that is quite unstable even in healthy children—is frequently not possible at all in children demonstrating deviating development or only marginally possible and very unstable. Due to the constant loss of balance, the child hardly moves its head at all, and sometimes blockage in the shoulder area is so marked that movement is not possible.

The hands are clenched into fists, the thumb is folded under and adducted at the basal joint. The position favors pronation. The hips are often still very flexed, a characteristic that is excessively noted in floppy children. The legs are in a frog position. No kicking at all or simultaneous kicking of both feet in an uncoordinated manner is noted. At times the child's legs merely lie on the surface, completely immobile and extended. There is very little mobility of the ankle joints, and the knees are hyperextended (Fig. **49**).

Fig. **49**

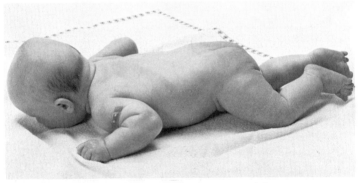

Pulling up from the supine position. From time to time, the child does not help at all or only very little when it is being pulled upward. The child's head is either "firmly fixed" into the shoulder area or hangs back floppily and then falls forward in an uncontrolled manner upon reaching the upright position.

There is a weak or complete lack of leg responses. Sometimes the knees are extended to such an extent that the child immediately assumes a "standing" position; hip flexion is difficult. When in a supported upright sitting position, the trunk is unstable. In cases of poor resting tone, the arms are either completely extended when the child is pulled up or hyperflexed.

If a sideways tilt occurs, the child's head falls downward and can scarcely be positioned horizontally (Fig. **50**).

Fig. **50**

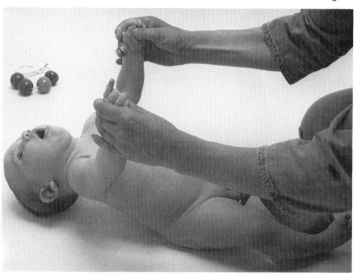

Setting the child on its feet while giving support under the armpits. The child does not put its weight down upon the pad; either there is too much flexion, or the child collapses (astasia). No slight cocontraction is noted, rather more a kind of positive, unmodifiable supporting reaction. There is very poor or inadequate head control. Trunk control can also only be described as mediocre to poor. The effort on the part of the examiner must be increased since the child does not help at all or only very slightly (Fig. 51).

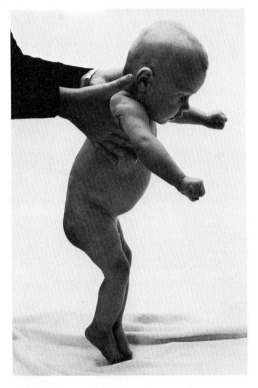

Fig. **51**

Reactions can be triggered intensely and persistently. Asymmetry should be looked for (physiological asymmetry should not be overlooked). When dealing with prematurely born children, such reactions are permitted to be triggered in a more prolonged and intense manner even considering the gestational age. All reactions that prevent coordination of movement should be considered as abnormal.

Fine Motor Function and Adaptation

Poor perception of persons and objects is evident. Initially, however, it must be ascertained to what extent this is due to sensory disturbances (disturbances of vision and/or hearing). A weakness in central processing may also be the problem.

The child does not follow objects sufficiently with its eyes. It is not yet capable of crossing over the midline since mobility of the head and the capacity to concentrate are limited.

The child's hands remain firmly balled even when they are touched; they remain in a fixed position and do not open.

Speech and Social Contact

Speech. Any utterances are either virtually nonexistent or barely perceptible. No cooing and squealing are heard. The child is "mute."

Crying may be undifferentiated, shrill, or whining. At times the child hardly cries at all and is very quiet and, therefore, quite inconspicuous to its environment.

Social contact. When the child is spoken to, it does not immediately smile and sometimes does not react at all. The child does not look at or fix its gaze upon the examiner; occasionally the same holds true for objects. All responses to unusual items in the environment virtually turn into catastrophes due to the child's inadequate reactions. It is difficult or impossible to pacify the child.

Posture and Muscle Tone

There are abnormal qualities of tone both actively in posture as well as passively during examination. Flexion or extension tone may prevail, or the tone may be changeable or so lax that the child is very unstable. When being felt, the joints seem either loosely hyperextensible or show increased tonus.

Coordination of movement is distinctly limited. Variations in tone become visible when checking shoulder and hip tension, and trunk flexibility is altered. Testing against resistance yields striking results.

Righting Reactions

Positioning of the head and body in space is very poor. The child should be examined in the prone and supine position, with sideways shift, and in the hanging position. The child does not adapt to changes of its position in space to a degree that is normal for this age.

Balancing Reactions

No stability is present when in the upright position. Adaption upon loss of balance does not occur. Any movement can trigger off displeasure, fright, or disquiet. When carrying out strong movements—which should only be tried if other, finer movements yielded no reaction—attempts toward adaption or changes in behavior frequently cannot be observed due to the fact that the child obviously is not able to perceive space.

Symmetry

The child may be symmetrical, or it may exceed the physiological proportions of an asymmetry. Since an asymmetry is recognizable in connection with any type of physical handicap, special significance should be attached to this. The most frequent sign that becomes visible is a scoliotic posture featuring a preference for one side through persistent tonic patterns of posture (ATNR).

Tonic Patterns of Posture, Reflexes, and Reactions of Early Infancy

Tonic patterns of posture can at times be very persistent and prevent any type of coordinated movement. The degree to which this holds true is important. Influences that do not prevent coordination are sometimes visible for a protracted period of time. They have little pathological significance.

The third month is a kind of transition period and decisions are more difficult to make; at this time it is the examiner's experience that plays an important role. Nonetheless, coordination of movement should be kept in mind.

It may still be possible to trigger reflexes and reactions beyond their respective period of development; their intensity may have increased, or they may occur asymmetrically. When dealing with prematurely born infants, one must take gestational age into consideration. Healthy yet prematurely born children often demonstrate such reactions longer or with greater intensity than is usual in healthy full-term infants.

Emotional Behavior

It is frequently not possible to get apprehensive, fidgety children into state 4 (according to Prechtl). All emotional reactions are exaggerated and inadequate. These children often do not calm down after being picked up, caressed, or spoken to, or through body warmth. Some of these children remain quiet only when they are with the mother and react inadequately to other persons.

At this age the mother-child relationship plays an important role and should not escape observation during examination. The examiner should place great value on this aspect. Problems should be solved by way of discussion if difficulties exist. The parents' fear of their child's possible handicap as well as not knowing whether or not a handicap exists render the situation very insecure. The effects thereof are reflected in the child's emotional behavior. It is best to examine children with conspicuous signs while they rest on the mother's lap.

3

Hearing and Localizing Sounds

A hearing test should be carried out, as it is necessary to exclude sensory disturbances when passing judgement on the child. Disturbances in central processing point to a different prognosis and require appropriate treatment.

During screening the child may show conspicuous signs; either it hears only loud noises, or it is unable to localize them properly. As a result, the child becomes quite irritated. This can be noticed in the child's behavior.

Sound Formation with Special Attention Given to Breathing, Sucking, and Swallowing

Sound formation appears to be an important topic since a child with increased or decreased basal tone has difficulty in articulating sounds. Imitation of its own noises is inadequate.

The manner in which the child cries gives the examiner information as to coordination within the phonation apparatus. Observation of breathing and the type of sucking and swallowing are of importance here.

It is important to question the mother, since she will most likely have noticed any difficulties that may exist. However, if she does not realize the significance of these difficulties, she might categorize the child as mentally handicapped.

The child's crying has a signaling effect and directs the mother's behavior.

Vision and Eye Movements

A child's inability to fix its gaze upon an object may point to a disturbance of the visual apparatus. However, it may also be due to disturbances in central processing. Limited motor ability impairs vision, because the eye, head, and neck muscles do not act in a coordinated manner. If there are any conspicuous signs, the child should undergo examination by an eye specialist. The neurological examination may be able to explain the striking aspects pertaining to motoricity. Weakness in central processing usually becomes noticeable at a later point in time and sometimes responds positively to stimulation by means of special education.

Grasping

At this early age, coordinated grasping is already in preparation. Irrespective of the fact that grasping includes kinaesthetic perception, the hand plays an important role. The way the hands are held and the positioning of the fingers in relation to each other gives information about the motor handicap. Objects are held either too tightly or too loosely. The child is frequently unable to look at the object, so it cannot recognize the object visually. The pathological pattern shows more or less clawlike fingers with turned-in thumbs which are adducted at the basal joint, making it impossible to use them for grasping. The hand is in pronation; the thumb and index finger are frequently more flexed than the other fingers.

The child is unable to make its hands meet at the midline; hand-eye coordination is either insufficiently present or not developed at all. As a result, sensory integration becomes more difficult.

Development

Since at 3 months of age the quality of future capabilities is being programed, the origins of many disturbances in cases of deviant development are laid down. The child—who does not consider itself to be reacting abnormally—develops inappropriate behavioral patterns adapted to the given situation by means of the capacities that the child actually possesses. Stabilization, which usually slowly takes place at this time, fails to occur. Consequently, exploration of the environment presents difficulties for the handicapped child. The consequences of such faulty development can be unbelievably severe and often remain throughout the child's entire life.

Fourth Month

Normal

Gross Motoricity

Supine position. The infant is able to lie symmetrically on its back and turn to both sides. Turning is carried out with a slight rotation. The child can hold its head at mid-position; however, one side is frequently preffered. Slight ATNR influences may still be in effect, but the child is consistently able to change its position. The child can lift its hands and join them at the midline and look at them; this series of movements is coordinated with head and body posture. The hands are open and the shoulders sometimes retracted, while the hands do not automatically close as a result. The child plays with its hands and is able to hold objects. The child already begins to put objects into its mouth. The object can be let go of, but this usually occurs involuntarily (Fig. 52).

Fig. **52**

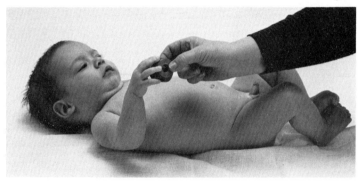

If an object is brought close enough for it to be seen by the child, mass movements sometimes occur before the child is able to stabilize itself in order to grasp the object.

The child's legs are outwardly rotated and abducted and kick alternatingly. The knees still demonstrate much flexion, but they can be extended. The feet are dorsiflexed, and the ankle joints are very flexible. When moving its head, the child will in rare cases demonstrate a Moro reaction sometimes only with open hands without abduction of the arms from the shoulder. As a whole, the movements appear somewhat more coordinated.

Prone position. The child can lie symmetrically on a surface; it lifts its head up to nearly 90°. The child supports itself quite sturdily on its lower arms.

The hands are sometimes still closed in this position but can easily be opened. The child does not yet attain complete balance in this position. Extension of the trunk and hip has advanced further. Preliminary crawling motion is evident. The child's legs are slightly outwardly rotated as well as abducted and kick alternatingly.

When the child's legs lie flat upon the surface, they are outwardly rotated and abducted. Its feet may be either dorsi-flexed or plantar-flexed. The ankle joints are flexible. From time to time swimming movements occur, but they are not the predominant pattern. The child's ability to extend itself is quite good (Fig. **53**).

Fig. **53**

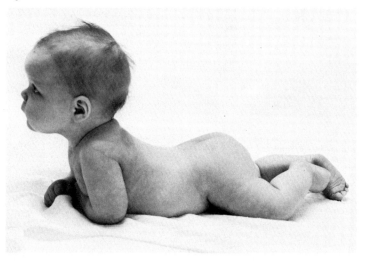

Pulling up from the supine position. The child helps the individual pulling it upward and demonstrates good head control. The legs are extended and only somewhat flexed at the knees. The child's head is stable and held in a midline position to the trunk.

When sitting, the trunk is not yet stable, and the back is hunched. If one holds the child at the trunk, the arms go into shoulder retraction. When the child is pulled upward by the hands, the arms are slightly flexed at the elbow joints. If one holds the child at its waist so that it leans sideways, the child adjusts its head to the new position in space, but it does not yet put its arms forward for support. Slight lateral asymmetry can be physiological (favorite side) (Figs. **54–57**).

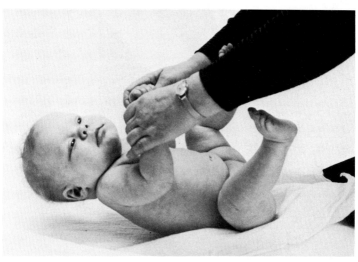

Fig. **54**

Fig. **55**

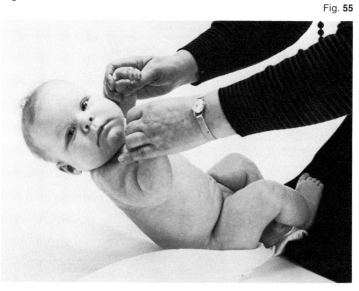

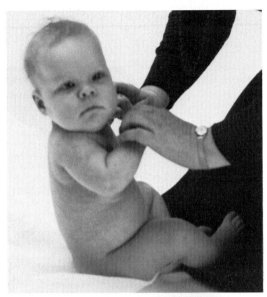

Fig. 56

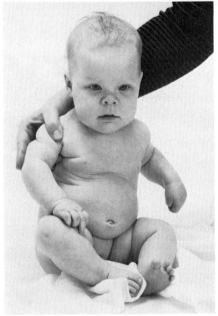

Fig. 57

Setting the child on its feet while giving support under the armpits. The child extends its legs toward the surface it is to be put down upon and a slight transfer of body weight occurs through cocontraction. The knees are extended, and the hips are flexed, while the trunk is extended. Head control is frequently already quite stable. Upon passive sideways tilting of the head, it usually properly adjusts to its position in space (Fig. **58**).

4

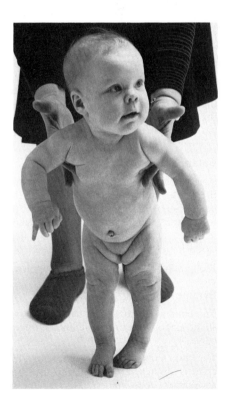

Fig. **58**

Posture and Muscle Tone

The child no longer demonstrates a constant flexor tone but instead is capable of attaining a certain amount of extension in every position. On passive examination, the child's tone is normal, sometimes a bit more lax and at other times a bit firmer, but always with a good amount of flexibility and without any limitations. As a result, the extremities are able to both flex and extend so as to allow for a coordinated sequence of movements. During examination, the child is able to hold its position as well as spontaneously move.

Passively moved extremities do not swing back into the original position; they either remain in the new position or are independently moved by the child. Joint mobility has improved. The joints already react in a dissociated manner. When movements occur on one side, there are also associated movements on the other side. The range of movement has substantially increased as compared with the previous month.

Righting Reactions

The child's head position is adjusted to any orientation the child may take up in space (test in the supine, prone, sideways, and hanging positions). The child already adjusts quite well to alterations of its position in space and demonstrates placing reactions of the body when the head is laid toward one side. The child's body then turns toward the opposite side. There are preliminary placing reactions of the body parts to the body.

Balancing Reactions

As a whole, the child has become somewhat more stable, especially in the supine and prone position. The sitting and standing positions are not yet stable. Nevertheless, whenever it loses its balance, it attempts to adapt its weight accordingly. The child succeeds at this as far as is feasible. The supporting reaction is not yet sufficient, but initially, extension of the arms without carriage of weight occurs.

Preliminary opening of the hands upon approaching a surface is noted.

Symmetry

The child is nearly symmetrical in all positions; there is sometimes a slight scoliotic posture while in a sitting position, but this can be overcome.

The child's favorite side is sometimes still very visible; however, if the child is stabilized, it frequently uses both hands. In cases of minor asymmetry, coordination of movement is uninhibited on both sides.

Tonic Patterns of Posture and Reactions of Early Infancy

Slight influences of tonic patterns of posture are sometimes still visible at this age (ATNR and TLR). However, coordination of movement is not impaired by this. The magnet reaction, Galant reaction, placing reaction, stepping and Bauer's reaction can no longer be elicited (when dealing with prematurely born children, gestational age should be kept in mind!). The palmar grasping reaction hardly exists anymore. The child usually reacts by briefly flexing its fingers; then it re-opens its hand. By contrast, plantar grasping reaction are easily elicited to equal degrees on both sides.

The Moro reaction should not occur any longer or only to a very minor degree. Sometimes during examination one sees a slight opening of the hands without any kind of further reaction of the rest of the body.

Fine Motor Function and Adaptation

The child perceives objects at the midline as well as beyond on both sides up to a distance of 20–30 cm. The child follows objects with its eyes as well as through head movements of more than 180°. It focuses upon an object and shows interest in it. It attempts to grasp the object.

The child's grasping movements are still very uncoordinated, not well directed, and quite abrupt as well as exaggerated. An object can be grasped, held, moved about, and let go of (unintentionally). However, the child carefully observes exactly what happens to its hand and the object it had been holding and tries to repeat the procedure with help from its mother. It obeserves its hands and its arm movements upwards, to the front, and to the side.

The child puts its fingers and objects into its mouth and sucks on them. The child shows resistance if a toy is taken away from it.

Grasping

The child is able to grasp objects held towards it with a palmar grasping motion; this movement is rather uncoordinated. There is still extensive pronation. If the child has the object in its hand, it clutches firmly and only lets go of it unintentionally. The child repeats the procedure during which time it sometimes watches the object. The child brings both hands up to the midline until the hands touch; at first this is unintentional, later it is intentional. The child plays with its hands. It puts toys into its mouth.

Speech and Social Contact

Speech. The child smiles when it is talked to; sometimes it even laughs out loud. It turns its head toward the speaking person and coos and squeals spontaneously. It enjoys hearing the noises it produces and repeats them. It turns toward noise sources and is very quiet and attentive. It tries to assert itself through crying and exhibits good voice modulation, already differentiated.

Social contact. It looks at the examiner and focuses its eyes upon that person. It precisely watches all faces directed toward it. If the child has a fearful mother, it can sometimes already demonstrate distinct reactions of being frightened of strangers or feeling uneasy. It can be pacified by being picked up, talked to, or caressed, and through body warmth.

Hearing and Localizing Sounds

When the child hears a noise, it becomes attentive. It can already distinguish different qualities of noise and prefers, for instance, music, singing, etc. One should test as many different types of noise as possible, such as a piping sound, a bell, a quiet voice, a loud voice, the sound of rustling paper. The child localizes the various directions from which the noises come and turns toward the source. The child seems to recognize repeated noises or even attempts to provoke their being repeated. It repeats the noises it produces itself.

Sound Formation with Special Attention Given to Breathing, Sucking, and Swallowing

The child enjoys hearing its own noises and repeats them. It cries loudly whenever it needs anything. Well-coordinated breathing, sucking, and swallowing.

Vision and Eye Movements

The child is able to focus well upon objects that are 20–30 cm away from it. It follows objects visually beyond the 180° mark (beyond the midline). The head also turns. Eye movements are coordinated, strabismus no longer exists. The child follows objects in all directions, toward the right, left, upwards, downwards (testing should take place with the child either sitting or lying on its back).

Emotional Behavior

The child should preferably be in state 4; deviations from state 4 must be distinctly documented. After a period of becoming accustomed to the new surroundings, the child smiles at the examiner. If the child has a fearful mother, it is likely to demonstrate a tendency toward being afraid of people it has never seen; however, the child can be pacified by being picked up, caressed, or talked to, and through body warmth. If this does not succeed, the examiner should let the child remain on the mother's lap during the examination.

Development

The child slowly becomes more stable, especially in the supine and prone position. The pattern of movement is modified, and extension improves. Body and head positioning in space is stabilized.

The result is that the child's relationship to its environment has improved; the child begins to explore its surroundings and seems mentally further developed than its motoricity would seem to allow. However, the child radiates signals to its mother that make it possible for her to react to her child's needs. Apart from its alimentary requirements and its need for sleep, the child also has the desire to make contact with its environment and to communicate. If the child does not succeed, it cries. The type of crying the child presents in this situation is demanding.

Deviating Development

Gross Motoricity

Supine position. The infant is often unable to lie symmetrically. The asymmetry frequently allows the child to turn only to one side, usually the poorer side, as the healthier one can more easily follow the turn. This is often caused by persistent tonic patterns of posture which impair coordination fo movement as they overlap (ATNR and TLR).

Shoulder retraction is accompanied by clenched fists, and the ability to bring hands together at the midline is missing. The capacity to grasp objects or put its fingers into its mouth is not possible to a normal degree.

Extension to a large or medium degree may be present, resulting in the opisthotonus position which the child cannot effectively overcome. There is an asymmetrical extension position of the thorax, with inward rotation and adduction patterns of the legs. Sometimes the legs are in a frog position or in a primitive position accompanied by flexion, but with no alternating kicking. The ankle joints are immobile or hyper-extensible, with few stereotyped movements.

The child rarely changes positions because, due to its stiffness or laxness, it is unable to attain an upright position against the force of gravity. In cases of hypertonia, extensor or flexor patterns are sometimes preferred (Fig. **59**).

Fig. **59**

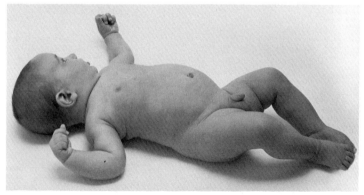

Prone position. A child's handicap frequently seems more obvious when the child is in a prone position because there it must perform more activities against the force of gravity (not possible in children demonstrating deviating development). Due to oversteering in cases of hypotonia, the child either does not raise its head well enough or raises its head excessively.

If the child's arms rest under its thorax, the child is unable to free them, and it cannot raise its head. The extent to which the child brings its arms forward of the shoulders shows to what degree the child is able to lift its head.

The child does not support itself on its lower arms to a sufficient degree as, at times, its arms are over-extended or unable to take the weight. The ability to balance, which is not yet sufficiently developed at this age anyway, is either only barely existent or virtually nonexistent. In this position, the child demonstrates a great amount of flexor tone or excessive extension, which makes it impossible for the child to adjust to a positon of balance. Numerous swimming movements are seen due to excessive extension. The legs are often immobile when in a frog position or extended, and there is no alternating backward kicking. The hip flexes all the more upon each movement of the head, hence making the child fall over forward. Extensive adduction of the legs is noted.

Upon loss of balance, the child's head is not adequately regulated in space; this is frequently due to blockage in the shoulder area. The fists are often clenched in pronation. The ankle joints are inflexible and hyperextensible (Fig. **60**).

Fig. **60**

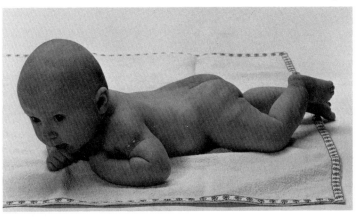

Pulling up from the supine position. When being pulled up and forward, the child does not help to a sufficient degree; its head falls backward or topples in a forward direction or sideways.

Sometimes the child's head does move upward with the shoulder area, but only because it is "walled into" that area and, therefore, not flexible.

When being pulled upward, the child is often stretched to such an extent that it goes directly into a standing position instead of a sitting position, and the hip cannot be moved. When sitting, the child demonstrates much instability accompanied by a lax and hunched back. Pathological asymmetrical posture accompanied by scoliosis is present. Either the arms are overextended, or the elbow joints are too flexed, while the child is being pulled upward.

If the child is tilted sideways, it does not extend its arms toward the surface, and its head is not sufficiently adjusted in space. The examiner must give the child excessive support in all positions (Figs. **61–63**).

Fig. **61**

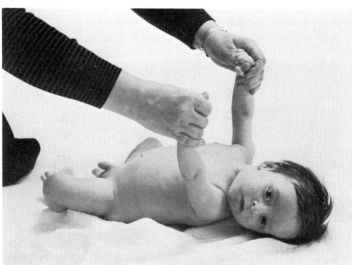

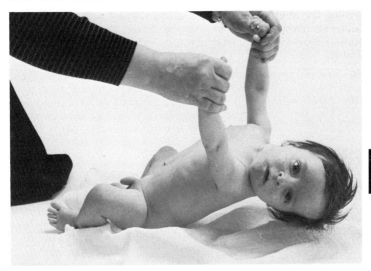

Fig. **62**

Fig. **63**

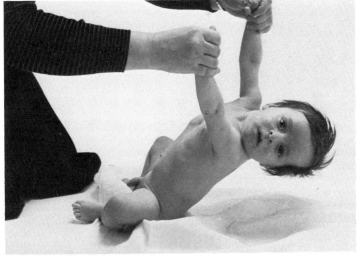

Setting the child on its feet while giving support under the armpits.
Upon being placed feet down upon the surface, the child does not put
its weight onto its feet at all or only to an insufficient degree. The child
collapses.

In cases of hypertonia the child only seems to stand. It looks like a
caricature of a child standing as the child is unable to alter its posture.
The child's entire body is extended, accompanied by a backward flexion. The arms are frequently very overextended or show shoulder
retraction. The child's head is displaced backwards (Fig. **64**).

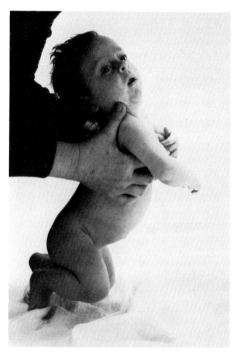

Fig. **64**

Reactions. All reactions that are generally only just visible at this age
and have slight influence may in some cases be very persistent (when
dealing with prematurely born infant, do not forget to consider the
gestational age). The extent of the persistence as well as asymmetry
are the most important indicators. Impairment of coordination of
movement must be noted. Here, the most significant aspect is the
quality of movement as well as to what extent the child is capable of
attaining an upright position against the force of gravity.

Fine Motor Function and Adaptation

After clarification of sensory modality disturbances (disturbances of vision or hearing), a child with poor visual perception must be examined with regard to the ability to focus upon persons and objects. A disturbance or weakness of the central processing system should be kept in mind. One observes whether the child does not visually fix objects or persons sufficiently. The child's glance wanders about without visually fixing any object. The child does not adequately react to stimuli.

If the child does manage to fix its glance on an object, it quickly breaks eye contact after only a brief period. The child easily becomes irritated by noise and light and promptly begins to cry. The child's cry is shrill and loud or whining but, in any case, signalizes discomfort.

4

Speech and Social Contact

Speech. Few sounds are produced; the child is very inarticulate. Its tongue is inflexible to such an extent that feeding difficulties arise. The child seems to be "mute." If the child's abnormalities are mainly located in its legs, sound and speech behavior may be completely normal.

Quiet children sometimes demonstrate a lack of sound formation. This should be considered abnormal. A child that constantly has an open mouth and shows signs of hypersalivation or difficulties in swallowing, sucking, or breathing must be attended to.

Social contact. The child may be conspicuous due to its lack of eye contact and of a spontaneous smile upon being spoken to. Sometimes the child more readily fixes its glance on objects than on people.

Difficult situations are responded to through inadequate reactions by the child; fear prevails. Sometimes it is difficult or even impossible to touch the child.

Posture and Muscle Tone

There are active as well as passive tone alterations. The child's tone may fall into the category of hypertonicity or hypotonicity, or alternate between them. Flexor or extensor tone may predominate. Coordination of movement may be disturbed; the joints either show too much tension or are overextended and unstable.

One must determine whether or not this could possibly be a variation of the norm in which there are phases of physiological instability during which the child's tone may be rather lax.

The tone should be considered abnormal if it does not allow for proper coordination. There is tension in the shoulder area, and trunk flexibility appears disturbed. When performing tests against resistance, there are deviations which reflect the quality of the tone.

True asymmetries should always be considered to be deviations. On the other hand, physiological asymmetries should not be misinterpreted.

Righting Reactions

Head and body adaptation to space is disturbed (the parents'/mother's handling techniques should be included in the examination, because these greatly influence the child's development). Righting reactions should be tested in the supine, prone, sideways, as well as hanging positions. All of the body's compensating movements should be precisely observed. A child with deviations in its motor development shows difficulty adapting to a change of position in space.

Balancing Reactions

Inadequate equilibrium is evident in all positions, especially supine and prone. At this age there are no balancing reactions in other positions. There is no adaptation to loss of balance. Any movement may elicit displeasure, fright, or disquiet. When performing more extensive movements—which should only be done if other more subtle movements do not bring forth reactions—movements of adaptation or changes in behavior frequently do not occur, because the child apparently does not perceive space.

Symmetry

A constant and recurring asymmetry should definitely be considered a deviation. Asymmetry appears to be of crucial importance in the recognition of central motor disturbances. Tonic patterns of posture (ATNR) show persistence. In the face of variations in tone and, hence, the inability to adapt to changing situations, asymmetry is inevitable.

Tonic Patterns of Posture and Reactions of Early Infancy

Persistent tonic patterns of posture which can be abruptly elicited by any movement of the head appear stereotypic. Coordination of movements is disturbed to a great extent, and the child is unable to restrain this. Minor tonic patterns of posture that can be overcome should be given attention, since they may be a sign of delayed development; however, they do not necessarily mean that a handicap exists.

Primitive reflex patterns should be viewed with this aspect in mind as well. In most cases they signal a delay in development. If they are asymmetrical, one should consider whether this is perhaps a motor disturbance (keep the child's gestational age in mind when dealing with prematurely born children).

Emotional Behavior

Easily frightened, restless children can hardly be brought into state 4. They either emotionally overreact or react inadequately. These children cannot be pacified by any manipulation, except perhaps by the mother.

The mother-child relationship should be observed during the course of the examination as there may already be disturbances there which, in turn, may supply further clues. The mother—who is just as dependent upon her child's emotions as vice versa—quickly notices any disturbances.

Any fear the mother may have when initially meeting the doctor has a repercussive effect on the child.

Peace and quiet during the examination eliminate many problems or bring them to light more readily. Allowing the child to remain on its mother's lap during the examination is often useful.

Hearing and Localizing Sounds

A hearing test should be performed in order to rule out the possiblity of a sensory modal disturbance. Weaknesses in central processing lead to a different prognosis and require treatment accordingly. During the hearing test (screening), it should be noted when the child does not direct its attention towards the source of noise or only inadequately reacts to noise, for instance, by loud crying. The child's behavior signals its irritation.

Sound Formation with Special Attention Given to Breathing, Sucking, and Swallowing

Depending upon the extent of the tone disturbance or handicap, aberrant sound formation is a particularly common characteristic. The child's ability to imitate its own noises is insufficient. The nature of the child's crying indicates that there may be disturbances in the coordination of the phonation apparatus. Breathing, sucking, and swallowing should be observed. Hypersalivation (excessive secretion of saliva, profuse drooling) may occur. Further information can be obtained by questioning the mother. The child's crying has a signaling effect upon the mother and directs her behavior.

Vision and Eye Movements

An inability in a child to fix its gaze upon a given object/person may be due to either impaired vision or a disturbance in central processing. In addition to the aforementioned, a motor disturbance accompanied by restricted head control or persistent tonic patterns of posture are sometimes the cause of visual impairments, since coordination of the senses and motoricity influences vision.

Grasping

If the child is not capable of approaching the midline with its hands, hand-eye coordination as well as coordinated grasping is unable to develop. Tonic patterns of posture and variations of tone result in the motor portion of grasping. If the shoulders are retracted, the hands balled, and the thumb adducted or folded under while the child is only able to hold its hands in pronation, it is very likely that the grasping process is disturbed.

If, in addition to the aforementioned, the child is unable to play using its fingers, thus making it impossible for the child to get to know its own body, disturbances in body image are certain to arise.

Development

During the course of the fourth month, a delay in development becomes quite obvious. Head and body stability is insufficient in the upright position. Complete extension or flexion patterns may dominate, thus making coordination of movements impossible or extremely difficult with regard to attaining a vertical position. Righting reactions are of considerable importance at this time. Distinct, pathological asymmetries should become visible by this age.

Mental development—which is closely linked to corresponding movements—shows elements of retardation which extend into the psychological area. The mother does not learn to help the child become more and more independent, because the child needs her too much, and she consequently misses the appropriate point in time. The child does not signal to the mother that she should omit certain types of support. The process of maturation of interaction between the mother and the child and, consequently, with the environment is severely disturbed.

Fifth Month

Normal

Gross Motoricity

Supine position. The infant is able to turn onto one side or the other from the supine position and occasionally onto its stomach. The infant touches its feet and puts them into its mouth. The infant touches its body; its hands are already open at this point. Sometimes the infant hyperextends its back, hence slightly lifting its hips which gives the impression of forming a bridge. The head is lifted up from the supine position, at which time the rest of the body is extended. Any objects grasped are put into the mouth and can also be released. The trunk is symmetrical in its alignment to the head. The legs are outwardly rotated and abducted. Frequently, alternating kicking is still noted, although sometimes only bending and stretching on both sides. The knees can be easily extended, and the ankle joints are mobile. Movements now seem more coordinated (Fig. **65**).

Fig. **65**

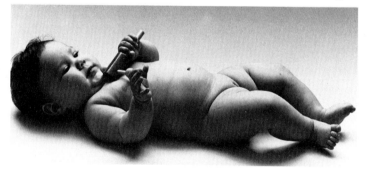

Prone position. The child lies symmetrically, the head can be easily lifted up to 90°, and there is good lower-arm support. There is a re-distribution of weight when in this position in order to release the other side and to stretch the arm forward. Rotation begins. There is no forward movement as yet. The legs are outwardly rotated and abducted. The hips lie flat on the underlying surface; the feet are dorsi-flexed or plantar-flexed and have mobile ankle joints. There are swimming movements due to initial extension. The head is moved from right to left and vice versa, and the infant fixes its gaze on objects (Fig. **66**).

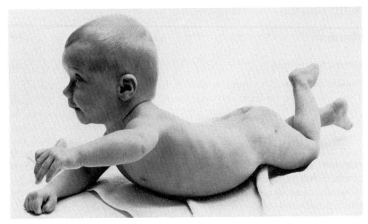

Fig. 66

Pulling the infant up from the supine position. The infant helps when being pulled up from the supine position; head control is quite good. The head can be pulled forward quite nicely and can then be turned to the side. The legs are extended while the infant is being pulled upward. The arms are bent at the elbow joints and are mobile (Figs. **67–69**).

Fig. 67

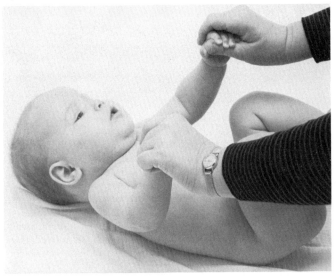

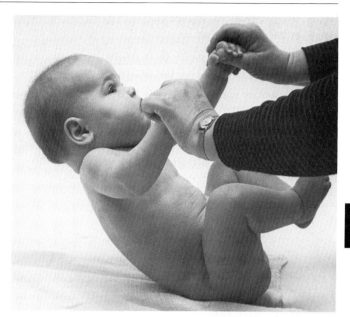

Fig. **68**

Fig. **69**

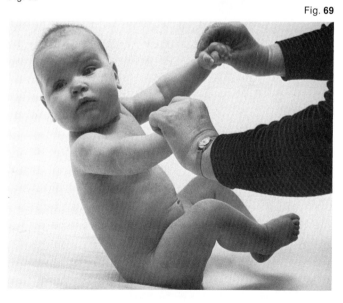

Sitting. Trunk stability begins to appear. The back is not yet completely extended, but it can be extended for a brief period of time. Shoulder retraction is a means of controlling balance. If the infant is held by the shoulders or at the waist, rotation with arms extended to the sides is initiated, but without taking up body weight.

The infant puts its arms forward as a means of support yet without complete assumption of body weight. The hips can be bent, and the legs are outwardly rotated and abducted and bent at the knees. The ankle joints are mobile. Good head positioning with respect to space is obvious. There is symmetrical trunk comportment or an occasional, slight physiological asymmetry that can be overcome (Fig. **70**).

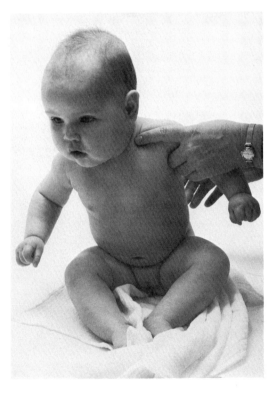

Fig. **70**

Setting the infant on its feet while giving support under the armpits.
The infant extends its legs toward the pad and takes up the body
weight upon bending at the hips. The knees are more flexible. Gently
guiding the infant with one's hands, one is able to feel the infant begin
to bob up and down (Fig. **71**).

5

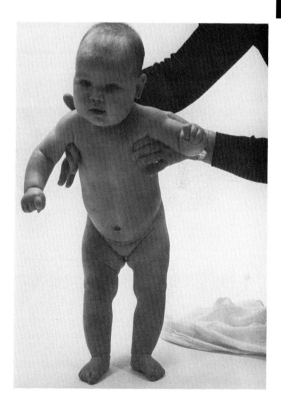

Fig. **71**

Posture and Muscle Tone

Muscle tone is normal in all passive tests; occasionally it is somewhat lax or somewhat firmer, but good mobility in all joints can be noted. A single tone quality is no longer predominant. Instead, there is a methodical ability to adjust the tonus in accordance with certain motor activities. The child is able to bend and stretch.

If a joint is moved passively, it no longer swings back into the original position but rather remains in the position it was in when released. The infant moves independently. Liberation of the joints from each other is considerably improved. There is still slight tension in the shoulder area. The hips are well abducted, but not excessively. The legs are easily extended; the ankle joints are very mobile. In passive tests, the range of movement is substantial. When the big toe is stretched, formation of the plantar arch can already be noted.

Righting Reactions

Head positioning with respect to space is good in all postures. There is a good righting reaction of the head with respect to the body and a beginning righting reaction of the body with respect to the body. There is the initiation of rotation as well as a Landau reaction (Figs. **72, 73**).

Fig. **72**

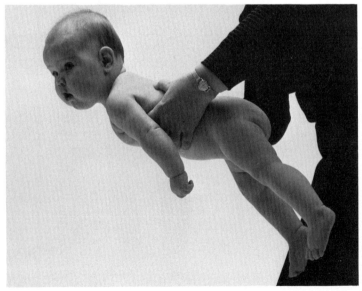

Balancing Reactions

The infant has become more stable in all positions, especially supine and prone. When sitting, the infant still displays trunk instability as well as a humpback. The hips are still bent excessively so that the infant falls forward. The ability to support itself on its arms and take on the body weight is quite good; nonetheless, the arms cannot yet be brought far enough forward to make complete support of the body weight possible since the hands are not yet open. The elbows are bent disproportionately. The child's parachute reaction is not yet good.

Symmetry

The infant is able to retain symmetry in all positions. The head and the trunk are balanced in mid-position. The child is able to pass from an asymmetrical to a symmetrical position. There are no limitations to coordination of symmetrical movements.

5

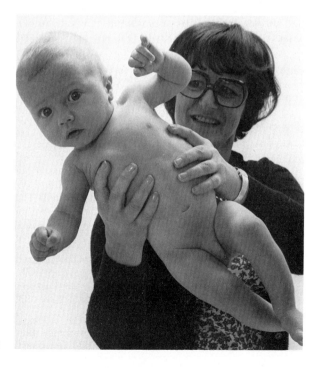

Fig. **73**

Tonic Patterns of Posture and Reactions of Early Infancy

Any tonic postural patterns as well as the Moro reaction and other primary reactions of early infancy have disappeared (in cases of the prematurely born, gestational age should be kept in mind). Should reactions appear, they only have pathological significance if they obstruct the coordination of movements. All these reactions are now restrained by more sophisticated centers of the brain; nevertheless, they are still components of the human motor system and become visible again in certain situations.

Fine Motor Function and Adaptation

If the infant is sufficiently stabilized, it is able to grasp for objects with both hands using the "entire palmar surface to grasp." The thumb is extended and slightly adducted. Toys are passed from one hand to the other, and the infant frequently puts them into its mouth. The infant plays with its feet, touches its body, and often puts its feet into its mouth. When sitting down firmly, it looks in an interested manner at objects which have been allowed to fall next to it. It observes larger and smaller objects, tries to grasp objects which are out of its reach, resists having toys taken away from it, and plays hide-and-go-seek.

The infant will eat a cookie without help that is placed in its hand. Sitting firmly, it will take a block in each hand. It can exchange the block from one hand to the other. Eye and head movements are more coordinated.

Grasping

Grasping still takes place with the palmar surface if the infant is stabilized. Pronation is no longer as considerable. The fingers are frequently open. Objects are held and only released unintentionally. Repetition occurs in accordance with the "trial and error" method. The infants looks at the objects it holds in its hands. The hands come together at the midline and touch. The infant plays with its hands.

Speech and Social Contact

Speech. The infant squeals and laughs and makes unarticulated noises. It stops crying when it notices music. It talks to itself. It produces new sound combinations such as ra, re, da, de, and go and begins to connect them, forming rhythmic chains of syllables like dadada or gegege.

Social contact. The child smiles at its mirror image and grabs for the bottle. It differentiates between a friendly and an earnest tone of voice as well as expression; it begins to seek contact by turning towards a speaking person. It ceases crying when spoken to. It differentiates between well-known and unfamiliar persons. At times it is afraid of strangers.

Hearing and Localizing Sounds

The infant hears well during all tests and turns toward the source of noise. Peace and quiet are important during examinations. It differentiates the quality of the sound depending upon the object being tested. It recognizes noises and may be thrilled by a certain noise while disliking another. It repeats its own noises and seems to like them; it even changes the key.

Sound Formation with Special Attention Given to Breathing, Sucking, and Swallowing

Phonation is good; details can already be noted. There is repetition and alteration of noises. The child cries loudly if it needs something or wants attention. There is considerable modification of crying depending upon what the child desires. Breathing is good.

Sucking und swallowing are well coordinated.

Vision and Eye Movements

The child is capable of fixing its gaze upon objects and adjusting its eye and/or head movements to them if it is in a suitable position. It follows objects with its gaze beyond the midline to 180°. There is no strabismus. Objects are followed at all levels (test in both the sitting and supine position).

Emotional Behavior

The infant tolerates establishing contact with an unfamiliar person after a certain period of time without being afraid if the mother motivates the infant to do so. This is not the case if the mother does not tolerate it.

The examining conditions which played such a significant role for observations previously are not as important for compiling results any more. If the infant's development is normal, the mother is generally so stable after 5 months that she can follow the doctor's examination of her infant with far less anxiety, which leads to a more peaceful atmosphere. A crying infant should be pacified by the examiner or the mother.

At times it is appropriate to examine the infant while it sits on its mother's lap.

If given words of encouragement, the infant smiles and sometimes grabs the examiner's hair—meaning that it is seeking contact and being playful. Various modes of behavior can already be noted at this age.

Development

The infant has become more physically stable, although it is still unable to execute coordinated movements when in an upright position (unstable phase of development). It tries to move against the force of gravity; head control has been improving consistently. There is an appearance of rotation and a good righting reaction. The child begins to explore its environment with its own means. There is an alert expression. The child cries whenever it needs or wants anything, and the way the child cries differs accordingly.

Sixth Month

Normal

Gross Motoricity

Supine position. The infant is capable of turning itself over from the supine into the prone position. It can do this to either side but usually prefers one side. It can touch its feet and its body in order to explore them. It can stretch its arms forward and raise its head. Occassionally it forms a "bridge" by extending its spine. The trunk is then lined up with the midline. The legs are outwardly rotated and show considerable abduction when bent; however, they can be easily extended. Hip abduction is good. Movements are more coordinated. The supine position is no longer preferred at this age (Figs. **74, 75**).

Fig. **74**

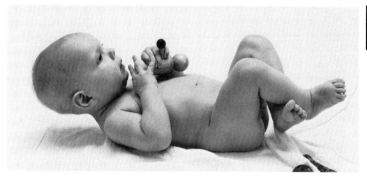

6

Fig. **75**

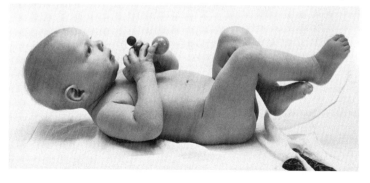

Prone positions. When in the prone position, the infant lifts its head considerably. Mid-position is 90°. The trunk is extended; the hips lie on the underlying surface.

The infant is able to support itself upon its lower arms and displays a good sense of balance (Fig. **76**). It redistributes its body weight onto one arm and slightly rotates and extends the other arm in order to grasp an object. Quite good rotation of the trunk is evident. The infant sometimes turns itself from its stomach onto its back. At first the child seems to "fall," although no longer en bloc but through rotation.

The infant produces "swimming movements" without obstructing its activity as a whole. Corrective movements are produced if it loses its balance. However, its sense of balance is good.

Fig. **76**

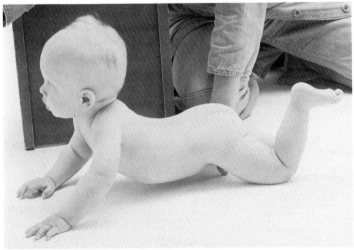

Pulling up into a sitting position. The child helps whoever is pulling it up if it receives enough stimulation. The infant actually wants to be in a sitting position, and it can prove difficult to get it back into the supine position. The infant displays good head control but sometimes only moderately good trunk control with a hunchback. When being pulled upward, the infant stretches its legs (Figs. **77–79**).

Sitting. If the infant is sitting, one can take away one's hands for a brief period. The infant support itself by leaning forward slightly but does not take enough up yet. Occasionally, the infant still enjoys throwing itself backwards which seems to be more of a request to play.

When sitting, the infant's legs are outwardly rotated, the hips are abducted, and the ankles are mobile. The infant sits with its back hunched and its knees bent. Support to the side is still insufficient. Upon shifting to the side, the arms are extended with good opening of the hands but with a remaining slight bend in the elbow joints. Thus, support of the body weight is not yet possible to a sufficient degree. Slight rotation remains. Posture is quite symmetrical.

6

Fig. **77**

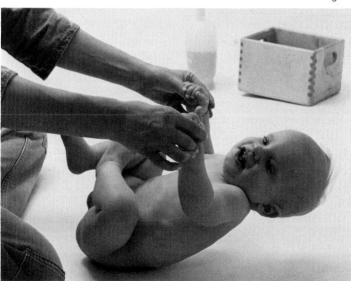

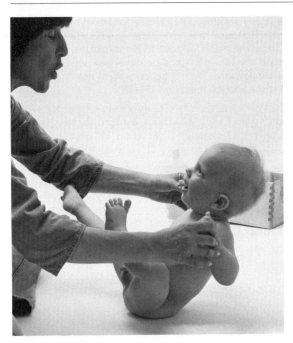

Fig. **78**

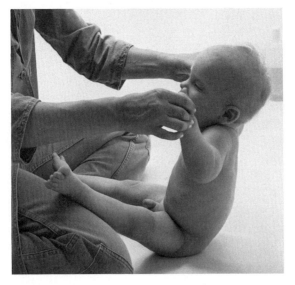

Fig. **79**

Pulling the infant up and setting it on its feet. If the infant is pulled up onto its feet, it distributes its weight quite well; however, one should not let go of it. The infant is not yet capable of holding itself. The knees are not rigidly recurved; they are merely in flexion. The child "bobs" up and down. It displays symmetrical posture and good head control, and the trunk is extended.

Should the child tilt sideways, it uses still inadequate corrective/compensatory movements to regain balance. The child positions its head with respect to gravity (Fig. **80**).

6

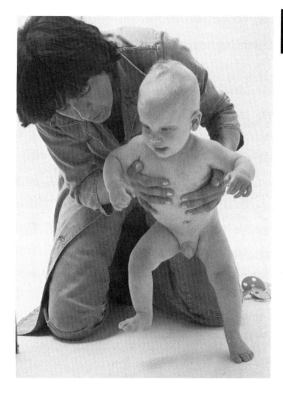

Fig. **80**

Posture and Muscle Tone

Muscle tone is normal. Since motoricity has become stabilized, tone also becomes stabilized, meaning it adjusts to the desired situation such as upright posture.

Functioning of flexion and extension becomes possible, as well as can be expected at this age. The joints become more independent. Posture maintenance improves and the transition to active motoricity accelerates. The first intermediate stages of movements become possible.

The tension in the shoulder area decreases, and the child learns to adjust its balance by using this area.

Hip abduction is good. All joints can be moved freely.

Righting Reactions

Head positioning with respect to the body is good as is the body's positioning with respect to the body. Whenever the child loses its balance, it adapts its movements, i.e. it catches itself when it falls.

Balancing Reactions

The infant's sense of balance is good in both the supine and prone positions but not yet as good as in the upright position. Nonetheless, the infant learns—albeit slowly at first—to improve its balancing reactions.

When sitting, the infant displays trunk instability, but with more extension and hence more stability.

Apart from the redistribution of weight for the purpose of regaining balance, support reactions also improve. When the infant tilts to one side, it stretches out its arms and opens its hands. Assumption of body weight when leaning forward is already quite good.

The infant's parachute reaction is good, its Landau reaction is very good, but extension is not quite complete.

Symmetry

Symmetrical comportment can be abandoned and assumed by the infant itself. There is initial preference of one hand for grasping.

Tonic Patterns of Posture and Reactions

Automatic and induced reactions are easily elicited and are the same on both sides. Tonic postural patterns or the primary reactions of early infancy can not longer be elicited (when dealing with prematurely born infants, keep gestational age in mind).

Fine Motor Function and Adaptation

If stabilized, the infant stretches out its arms and hands and grasps objects. The objects are then clasped; the thumb is already held in certain opposition thereto, but it is still somewhat adducted at the basal joint. If the infant wishes to pick up small objects, it still uses the entire surface of the palm (palmar grasping). Toys are passed from one hand to the other over the midline. Occasionally the infant still puts objects into its mouth.

The infant follows falling objects with its gaze, stretches toward objects that are outside of its reach, and picks up objects with both hands at the same time. The infant uses the "flat-nosed pliers grasp" to pick up small objects.

The infant eats crackers, plays hide-and-seek, and objects when toys are taken away from it.

Grasping

If the infant is stabilized, it grasps for objects outside of its reach. At times, it wishes to grasp while lacking the motor requirements to do so.

6

Its hands are opened and its fingers considerably well prepared for finer activities. The infant looks at what it picks up. Its hands meet at the midline; it plays with its hands and feet. It touches and learns to tell the difference between materials. Here, it first only differentiates between pleasant and unpleasant surfaces. The resulting reactions are contentment and discomfort.

Speech and Social Contact

Speech: The infant "talks" even when alone. It produces new sound formations such as ra, re, da, de, and go and joins them together to make rhythmic chains of syllables like dadada, gegege. It says Mama and Papa very spontaneously and for no apparent reason and begins to imitate sounds. It laughs and squeals loudly.

Social contact: The infant is shy when it sees unfamiliar faces but is not always afraid. It laughs if coaxed to do so and, after it has become accustomed to the examiner, it laughs whenever its mother laughs. The infant laughs at its mirror image and differentiates between a strict and loving tone of voice; it notices changes in facial expression and reacts to them. It turns toward sources of noise and reacts adequately to both pleasant and unpleasant situations.

Hearing and Localizing Sounds

The infant turns toward a noise source and can discriminate the quality of the noise.

The infant responds to loud, shrill noises with discontent and listens attentively to noises pleasing to it. It hears noises made by itself and repeats them.

Sound Formation with Special Attention Given to Breathing, Sucking, and Swallowing

Good phonation appears which makes nuances recognizable. The infant cries loudly whenever it needs anything or desires attention. There is significant modification of crying noises depending on the purpose. There is good breathing; sucking and swallowing are well coordinated.

Vision and Eye Movements

The infant follows people and objects with its gaze. It looks at everything, even what it has in its hand. There is good hand-eye coordination. Everything is followed at various levels. There is no strabismus (examine infant while lying on back and sitting).

Emotional Behavior

The infant takes up contact with its environment quite readily. If attention is turned to the infant, it reacts in a positive manner if the mother joins in. Contentment and discomfort are made known.

A crying or screaming infant can be easily pacified or distracted by a skillful examiner or by the mother. The infant smiles at strangers, nonetheless at times with a quiet, yet skeptical expression. It is very curious and enjoys exploring its surroundings. The infant is grateful for any kind of help as long as this is given adequately. It tries to attract attention (using all the means it possesses).

Development

This month seems to be a very decisive point in the infant's development. The upright position becomes more and more stable, and there is more balance in both the supine and prone positions. Changes of position broaden the infant's horizon; it has already become much more interested and curious.

Head control is good, rotation improves, and thus the infant's motoricity is able to function better. It begins to process perceptions and to categorize them. Visual, acoustic, and tactile-kinesthetic perception are based upon motor functions. The infant takes up contact with its environment very easily.

Seventh Month

Normal

Gross Motoricity

Supine position. The child no longer remains in the supine position. It turns over immediately and is able to do so from both sides. It is able to stretch its arms and raise its head so as to signal that it wishes to be picked up. As soon as it is touched, it pulls itself upward with almost no help. No dominant stretching or bending pattern is present (Fig. **81**).

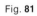

Fig. **81**

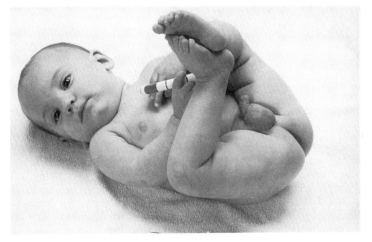

Prone position. When in the prone position, the child raises its head well. It redistributes its weight and pulls its legs up under its stomach in order to attain an upright position but falls back into the prone position. The child continuously repeats whatever it has been practicing. It turns itself on its own axis in this position and moves backwards if it tries to move forward. It extends one arm if it wishes to touch an object. Occasionally, the child stretches its arms and supports itself with extended elbow joints. The child's posture is symmetrical.

The hips lie directly upon the underlying surface, while the legs are abducted and slightly bent and mobile in all joints (Fig. **82**).

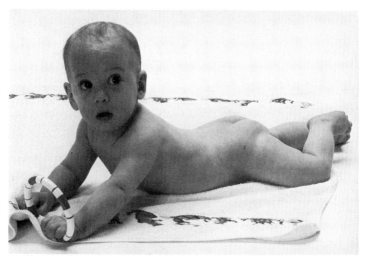

Fig. **82**

Sitting. Now, when the child is pulled up into a sitting position, it seems more stable. It is readily able to support itself through weight distribution when tilted forward. Upon passive sideways tilting, the child stretches its arms and hands and assumes its own weight. Rotation is not yet good. The child displays a hunchback, but it can be stretched quite considerably. Its legs are abducted, and the hips are bent properly (Figs. **83, 84**).

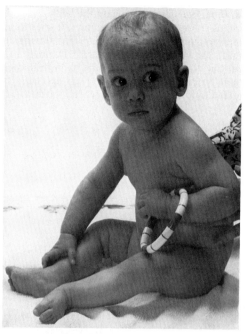

Fig. **83**

7

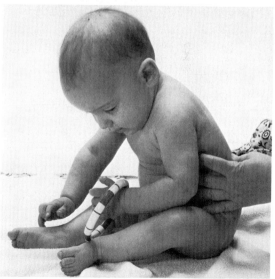

Fig. **84**

Rolling, creeping, moving on the belly. Since the child is not yet capable of standing firmly on all fours, it tries to move forward by rolling and sometimes even by crawling and moving on its belly (for the most part, the child slides backwards) in order to, for example, reach a certain object. In doing so, the child displays considerable stretching activity. Frequently, it pulls its legs up under its stomach and achieves a kind of forward movement when it pushes its legs out again (Fig. **85**).

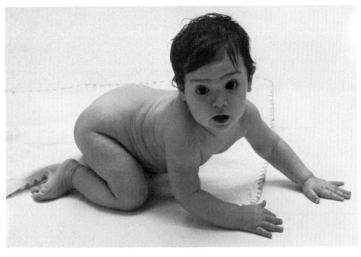

Fig. **85**

Setting the child on its feet while giving support under its armpits.
When the child is placed on its feet in this manner, it assumes its body
weight and bobs up and down in this position. For a brief period, the
child assumes its entire body weight.

The hips are already well extended, but in their entirety they are quite
flexible. If the child tilts to one side, it undertakes corrective/compen-
satory movements; there is good head positioning with respect to
space. Symmetrical posture is present (Fig. **86**).

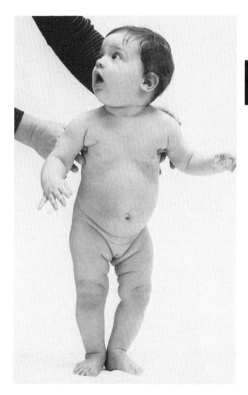

Fig. **86**

Posture and Muscle Tone

Tone is normal, and therefore, the motor system has become more stable. The child's tone can become accustomed and adjust to different situations. Posture maintenance becomes more secure. The intermediate stages of movements improve. There is good hip abduction and good mobility in all joints.

Righting Reactions

There is good head positioning with respect to space. Righting reactions of the head with respect to the body and of the body with respect to the body are considerable. If the child loses its balance, it adjusts to the new situation by way of good righting reactions with respect to gravity (Figs. **87, 88**).

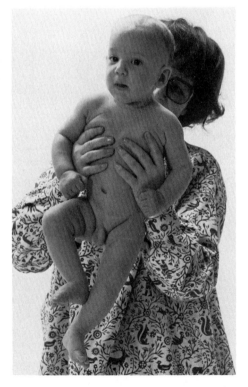

Fig. **87**

7

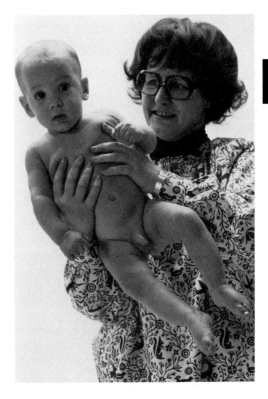

Fig. **88**

Balancing Reactions

The child displays good balance in both the supine as well as the prone position; there are initial signs of balance in the sitting position. The child achieves improvements in balance every day, and it tries to find out how far it can get. When the child moves, adjustment of balance takes place through regulation and counterregulation. The support reactions help here. There is a parachute reaction and a fairly good Landau reaction (Figs. **89–91**).

Fig. **89**

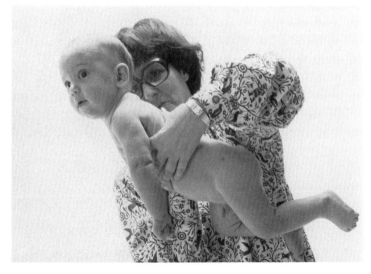

Fig. **90**

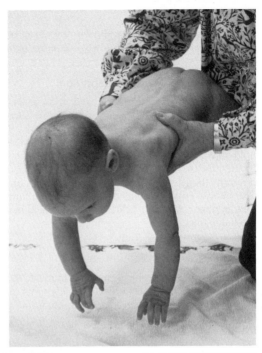

7

Fig. **91**

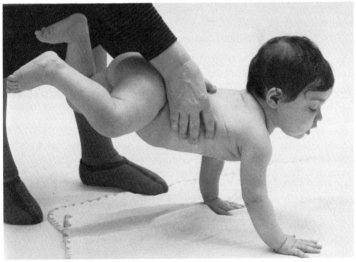

Symmetry

The child displays symmetrical posture that can be altered. There is no constant posture. One hand slowly becomes dominant.

Fine Motor Function and Adaptation

The child reaches for objects and tries to stabilize itself for this purpose. However, it does not as yet always succeed. Small and large objects are grasped—for the most part with the palmar surface—completely. The "flat-nosed pliers grasp" is still in use. The child is able to hold objects simultaneously in both hands and play with them. It learns to identify two objects by knocking them together, and it tries out different things. It can pass the objects from one hand to the other. The child's grip is usually made up of its thumb, index finger, and middle finger. More intricate objects are held between the thumb and the index finger.

Grasping

The child reaches for objects in a continuously more coordinated manner. It even tries to grasp objects outside of its reach. The child's eyes appear to want more than is possible according to its motor development. Its hands are open, and the fingers are prepared for finer movements.

The child looks at the object it grasps. Its hands meet at the midline; it plays with its hands and feet. It touches objects and learns to discriminate between pleasant and unpleasant surfaces and materials. The child's reactions are either pleasure or discomfort.

Speech and Social Contact

Speech: The child speaks its first syllables such as mama, dada, papa. It imitates sounds and loves to "talk" a lot. The child repeats its own sounds.

Social contact: Looking at another person is a form of "speaking"; hence, the child first takes up contact with a person through "eye contact." The child enjoys recognizing people it has seen before. Strangers are looked at skeptically. The child seems somewhat shy, but not necessarily afraid. It enjoys seeing its mirror image. It listens attentively and reacts according to the tone addressed to it (whether strict or friendly), displaying either pleasure or discomfort. It turns toward a source of noise and reacts in an adequate manner to pleasant or unpleasant situations.

Hearing and Localizing Sounds

The child listens attentively when it hears a noise and turns toward the source of the noise. The child responds to unpleasant noises with discomfort. It hears noises it makes itself and imitates them. The child also imitates noises from elsewhere.

Sound Formation with Special Attention Given to Breathing, Sucking, and Swallowing

There is good phonation with nuances as well as repetition and alteration of sounds. The child cries loudly and quietly; this shows its desire to communicate. The sounds are modified to suit its need. There is good breathing and sucking; swallowing is well coordinated.

Vision and Eye movements

Coordination of the eye muscles is already good. Hand-eye coordination is good; the child looks at objects and people. It looks at the objects it holds in its hands. The child follows whatever it is looking at with its eyes at all levels. There is no strabismus.

Routines of Daily Life

The child eats cookies if they are handed to it. It begins to drink from a cup that is held for it and eats from a spoon. The child does not slobber much any more.

Emotional Behavior

The child increasingly takes up contact with its environment in a lively manner and not merely unselectively. It begins to chose the people it likes. At this age, the child also begins to bring about situations it desires by way of rather skillful tactics; for example, through a certain mode of crying (demanding), it gains its mother's attention.

The child is curious and enjoys discovering its surroundings. It is grateful for any help that is geared towards its needs.

Development

Further stabilization and socialization take place. The child broadens its horizons through better motoricity. Curiosity becomes the child's motive for improving stabilization. Improved motoricity gives the child what it requires in order to be able to explore its surroundings. There is good head control, improved rotation, and balance.

Visual, acoustic, tactile, and kinesthetic qualities of perception are integrated. The child is good at taking up contact with people and in differentiating between people who are familiar or strangers to it.

Eighth Month

Normal

Gross Motoricity

Supine position. The child does not remain in this position, but rather turns over into the prone position from both sides (Fig. **92**).

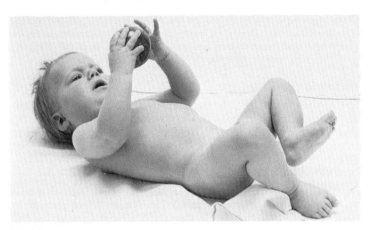

Fig. **92**

Fig. **93**

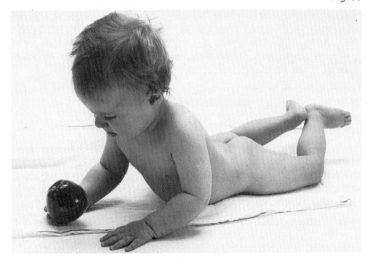

Prone position. Good head control and extension are evident. The child is capable of entering into the crawling position through bending patterns. Occasionally the child even crawls, although it is insecure and lacks rotation. It turns in a circle around its own axis.

The hips are outwardly rotated and the legs easily movable. The child achieves the sitting position—at times with help—by way of the prone position and on its side. It still frequently moves about on its belly (Fig. **93**).

Sitting. When the child sits, it is capable of supporting itself on the sides and here displays quite good rotation. Its back is straight, and trunk control is good, as is head control. The child turns around its own axis. All movements appear to be coordinated (Fig. **94**).

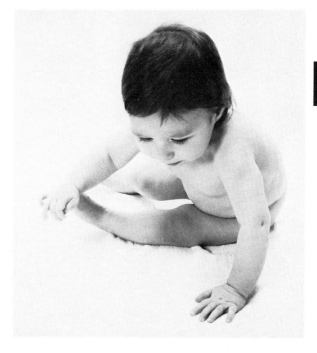

Fig. **94**

Pulling up into a standing position. The child pulls itself upward using the examiner's hand. Occasionally, the child uses objects for this purpose if they are very stable. The child then stands, slightly bobbing. The toes are clawed, since the child's balance is not yet very good in this position. The grasping reflex is still visible in the feet (Fig. **95**).

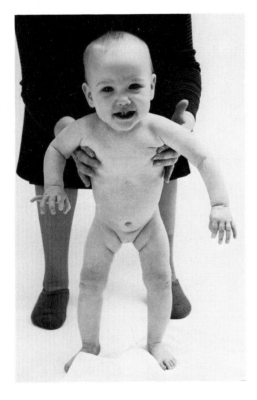

Fig. **95**

Crawling. The child enters into the crawling position; it crawls with still somewhat inadequate rotation. However, at this age, some children learn this very quickly.

Now and then, the child enters the sitting position by way of rotation into a sideways sitting position and then onto the actual sitting position. It is able to leave these positions very quickly. There are numerous movements. The child enjoys being able to move itself forward and does this so extensively that its environment must constantly be wary (Fig. **96**).

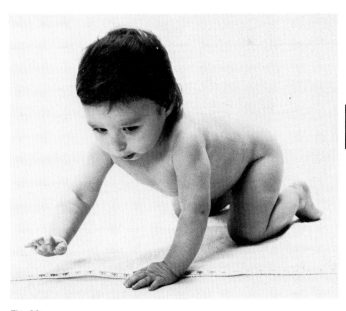

Fig. **96**

8

Standing. Standing is only possible if the child is given some support. Nonetheless, the child supports its body weight to a certain degree and bobs up and down. If it lets go, it tries again and again to pull itself up, especially if it is trying to reach something (Fig. **97**).

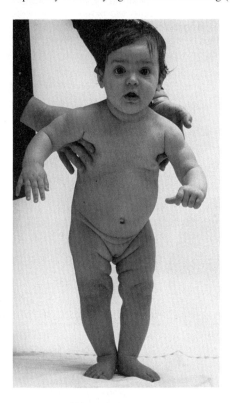

Fig. **97**

Posture and Muscle Tone

The child displays normal tone and should soon attain sufficient stability to be able to support the upright position. When doing a passive check, the child's joints are all very mobile if the child allows itself to be touched.

The child's active movements are good, and posture retention hints at a physiological, not yet quite stabilized tone. The child's ability to maintain posture is not yet complete; there is improvement in the intermediate stages of movements. There is good abduction of the hips and good mobility in the joints.

Righting Reactions

There is good head positioning in space. The righting reactions of the head with respect to the body and of the body with respect to the body are distinctly visible. Upon loss of balance, the child adjusts to the new situation through good righting reactions (Figs. **98, 99**).

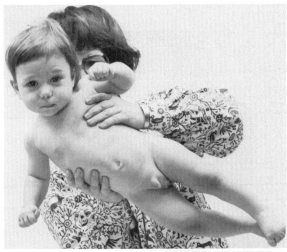

Fig. **98**

8

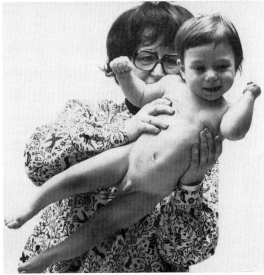

Fig. **99**

Balancing Reactions

There is a good sense of balance in the supine and prone positions; the child begins to sit. There is constant improvement of balance; the child is always trying things. In cases of loss of balance, regulation and counter-regulation have improved. Supporting reactions, parachute reaction, and the Landau reaction are good (Figs. **100, 101**).

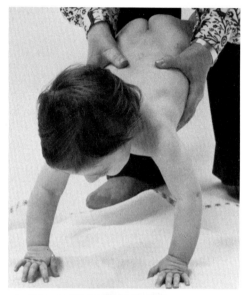

Figs. **100, 101**

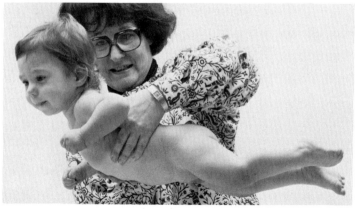

Symmetry

The child is able to abandon any asymmetrical posture and return to a symmetrical one. There is a distinct hand preference, although the child still uses both hands a lot.

Fine Motor Function and Adaptation

The child reaches for two dice with one hand. If one of the dice has already been grasped, it is held in such a manner that the child can also pick up the second one. The child reaches for toys within its grasping range. It attempts to grasp all toys within its reach. It looks at toys that have fallen, claps its hands together, and waves "bye-bye" if prompted to do so. It plays hide-and-seek.

The child intentionally drops objects that it has been holding between its index finger and thumb. It plays with small and large objects on the table and tries to find out what happens if it pushes them or throws them down. If the child throws an object down and its mother picks it up, the child will repeat this little game until the mother gives up.

Grasping

The child reaches for objects in the supine, prone, and stable sitting position. It attempts to grasp objects outside its reach. Its hands are open, and its fingers are prepared for finer movements.

The child looks at what it has picked up, its hands meet at the midline, and it plays with its hands and its feet.

It feels and touches objects and becomes acquainted with various materials. It learns to differentiate between pleasant and unpleasant surfaces. The child displays reactions of either pleasure or discomfort, depending upon which type of surface it has touched. It picks up small objects with its thumb and index finger; the "flat-nosed pliers grasp" is still apparent. Supination is easily possible, and the shoulders are almost completely movable at all levels. The child is able to stretch forward.

Speech and Social Contact

Speech. The child speaks its first double syllables such as Mama, Papa, dada, tata. It imitates its own sounds an others that it hears. It enjoys "talking" profusely.

Social contact. The child takes up contact with its environment through expressions, smiles, and nice-sounding noises that have a pacifying effect on the child. It looks at strangers very skeptically and, in this month of life, frequently seems afraid of them. It is not yet known with certainty to what extent the child's "being afraid of strangers" is part of the development process as a whole or is a characteristic only in certain children.

Hearing and Localizing Sounds

The child listens attentively when it hears noises and turns toward their source. It differentiates the quality of the noises. It hears its own sounds and imitates those from elsewhere.

Sound Formation with Special Attention Given to Breathing, Sucking, and Swallowing

There is good phonation with nuances and repetition and alteration of sounds. The child cries both loudly and quietly in order to make itself understood. The child makes sounds that resemble talking. Breathing is good; sucking and swallowing are coordinated.

Vision and Eye Movements

There is good coordination of eye muscles. Hand-eye coordination is already considerable. The child looks at objects as well as at people. It looks at the things it is holding in its hands. It watches objects at all levels. There is no strabismus.

Routines of Daily Life

The child eats cookies if they are handed to it. It will drink from a cup that is held in position for it and eat from a spoon at feeding time. Some children will allow themselves to be set on a potty, but there is as yet no bladder control.

Emotional Behavior

The child choses the people with whom it would like to have contact. If it feels afraid, it will cry. However, the mother is no longer the only person the child relates to. It reacts to "no" or to approval. It tries to achieve desirable situations through skillful tactics. The child finds out weaknesses in its parents. Much curiosity is evident; the child enjoys discovering new things. It is thankful for any help it can get in achieving whatever it desires so long as this help is related to those desires.

Development

The child is now much more stable in the upright position, although still a bit shaky. In this position, the child is also mentally better able to discover its surroundings. Permanent movements, alterations of position, and the continuous attempt to reach something within its range of view are the factors that now determine the child's development.

The child enjoys learning and includes its environment in this process. The mother receives signals that let her know the child wants her present at all times. The child learns all the tricks that cause the people in its environment to help it to broaden its field of activity.

Deviating Development

Motoricity

Supine position. It should be considered suspicious if the child remains lying on its back and does not turn over onto its stomach. Furthermore, one must find out whether the child is able to turn over from both sides or whether it prefers one side excessively (Fig. **102**).

Fig. **102**

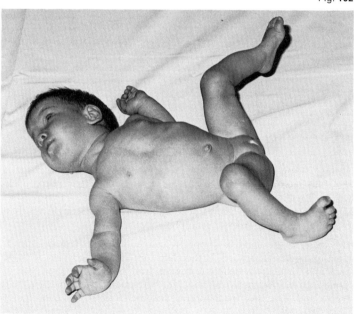

8

Prone position. Inadequate or poor head control and either poor or excessive extension is obvious. In such a case, transition to the crawling stage is distinctly impeded. There is abnormal moving about on the stomach. The hips are not well abducted in cases of hypertonicity, and in cases of laxity, they are too strong and unstable in function. There are few or excessive leg movements. Both the hypertonic and lax child displays insufficient mobility. A child with alternating tone displays excessive mobility (Fig. **103**).

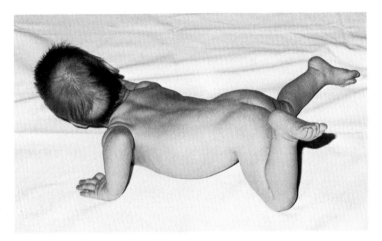

Fig. **103**

Sitting. When sitting, the child displays inadequate stability. Should the child have an impediment of bending in the hips that pulls it backwards, it will lean forward in an attempt to compensate, thus producing a hunchback. The child's head cannot be lifted straight up. It is brought forward in order to retain balance.

However, if the child is floppy, it cannot hold itself in an upright position and falls forward. It the child has alternating tonus, it sways back and forth and is unable to remain firm. Support through arms or hands can be obstructed by shoulder retraction, fist formation, bent arms, and excessive pronation. Movements are not coordinated (Figs. **104–106**).

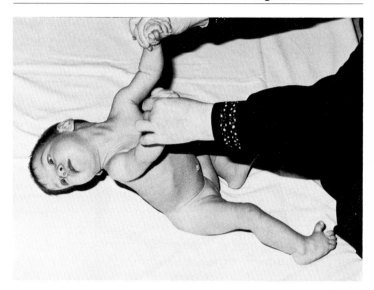

Fig. **104**
Fig. **105**

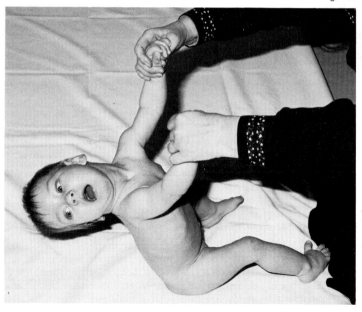

8

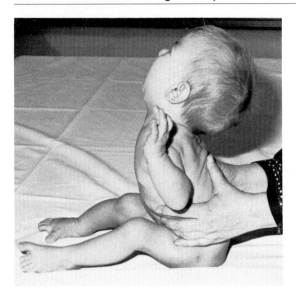

Fig. **106**

Pulling up into a standing position. The child does not yet help when it is being pulled into a standing position. The arms are either excessively bent or stretched at the elbow joints. The child does not take on the load of its body weight when it is set on its feet. Either the equinus position or excessively floppy ankle joints prevent this. The child's toes are rounded like claws. A grasping foot reflex is still very apparent (Fig. **107**).

Crawling. Crawling is not yet possible. Occasionally the child can manage to stand on all fours for a short period if it is put into that position. The sideways sitting position is sometimes assumed by the child, but on one side only and with poor rotation that lacks stability.

Standing. The child is unable to stand even if it is supported. When the child attempts to stand, its hips become excessively bent, and its knees recurve. Sometimes astasia is obvious.

Posture and Muscle Tone

The child's basic tone is either hypertonic, hypotonic, or alternating, hence influencing stability in the upright position. Mobility of the joints is altered. Posture and the retention thereof are impaired. Intermediate stages of movements are not easy. Hip abduction and adduction are altered. In children with persistent tonic posture patterns, the

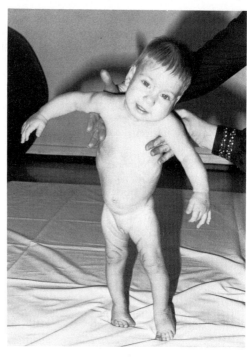

Fig. **107**

8

distribution of tone throughout the muscular system is influenced, thus strengthening alterations in tone.

Righting Reactions

The child's righting reactions are either inadequate or poor. Head positioning with respect to gravity is unstable. The child's head is uncontrolled and falls forwards, backwards, or sideways. Children that are mainly laid on their stomachs can frequently hold their heads better coming from this position than pulling upward from the supine position. The righting reactions of the body with respect to the body are not good enough to maintain an upright position. The child displays poor compensation when it loses its balance.

Balancing Reactions

There is poor sense of balance in both the prone and supine positions and consequently, balance is also poor in the sitting position. There is poor regulation and counterregulation on loss of balance. Parachute reaction and the Landau reaction are either insufficient or nonexistent.

Symmetry

The child is unable to return to a symmetrical position after having been in an asymmetrical one or it consistently prefers one side, whereby the other side is not even taken notice of. The unattractive side may be more affected at the arms and hands or legs and feet. The child hardly even looks at that side and rarely reaches for its body or objects with the affected hand.

Fine Motor Function

There is no coordinated grasping which is sometimes only conspicuous in one hand. The child does not look at the objects it wishes to grasp. Its hands are often still fisted, pronated and lying next to its body. The child sometimes does not even take notice of it. If the child does grasp and even perhaps looks at an object, the grasp is very inexact. Rarely is the child successfull in this endeavor and soon gives up trying. The child carries out no activities in which both hands come together at the midline such as waving "bye-bye" or clapping. It does not try to find out if it is able to grasp an object. If the child does have an object in its hand (e.g., by way of the grasping reaction), it does not release the object. It does not watch falling objects and appears uninterested. The child's gaze seems to wander about, never remaining set on one item for any length of time. Hence, it does not fix its gaze on anything. If the child does manage to fix its gaze on something, the object disappears from the child's gaze quickly, and the child appears not to be concentrating. Objects the child wishes to have or sudden noises and light frequently seem to be discomforting. It is unable to adapt to changes and, due to this, becomes unhappy. It cries in a shrill or whining voice to signal discomfort. Other children no longer seem to become irritated through such abnormalities and give up. They turn their attention to new activities extremely quickly; however, should they experience the same failure in this new activity, they also respond by showing their displeasure.

Grasping

Since these children are not stable in any type of upright position, they have great difficulty grasping anything they aim for (this especially holds true for floppy children). When movements are sluggish or tonic posture patterns exist, the child gives up trying to grasp. In such cases, any mobilization seems frightening to the child and results in panic. Objects outside of the child's range cannot be reached, because the child is too unstable and unable to free itself of the stiff patterns of movement. Inadequate righting and balancing reactions increase the child's discomfort.

The child's behavior appears to be inadequate. This is because the child lacks a proper feeling for space and is merely able to gather tactile experience insufficiently. It does not learn to recognize objects through grasping and processes signals incorrectly so that its reactions seem "wrong" to its environment.

When grasping for an object, the child does not possess adequate regulation so that its hold is either too weak or exaggerated. Hence, materials are not categorized properly, and differentiation is almost impossible.

If signals are incorrectly received, the reactions cannot be true responses to the given situation. Interaction with the environment becomes a misunderstanding and, consequently, more confusing. The child signalizes discomfort.

The child is not capable of grasping small objects and, therefore, experiences continuous failures. Some children give up. This makes them appear to be mentally impaired, although they would display normal developmental patterns if their motor system were intact.

The child is frequently unable to look at the object it would like to grasp, meaning that hand-eye coordination has not developed or insufficiently so. The child is unable to develop a feeling for space, as this implies stereoscopic vision. Objects do not stand out from their backgrounds for the child. Agnosia and, later, apraxia may arise.

Speech and Social Contact

Speech. If the child displays disturbances in mouth coordination, it is unable to pronounce the initial double syllables. Expressive language is prevented. The child is readily able to learn by hearing and later has a good understanding for language/speech, yet it is not able to form the sounds, and imitation of its own sounds is inadequate. As there is frequently an increase in tongue tone, no sounds are produced, and the child appears mute.

Social contact. Due to the child's insufficient fixation, it has no contact with its environment. The child's gaze wanders about restlessly and is still not constant enough to take up contact with the person to whom it relates. These children sometimes appear blind. Should the child—in addition to the aforementioned—have inadequate visual-learning capabilities, the people around it frequently conclude that the child is mentally handicapped and displays autistic characteristics. Special attention should be paid to this point in children with poor head control or considerable instability when in an upright position.

Children who are excessively afraid of strangers or are too trusting toward them should be carefully observed. The mother is very sensitive toward this characteristic and is often able to express it distinctly. One should listen very attentively to her whenever she talks about this point. Light or noises do not prompt the child to react accordingly but rather produce discomfort or indifference.

Hearing and Localizing Sounds

The child does not immediately turn toward a noise source although one can be certain (after having had the child tested by an ear specialist) that it is able to hear. Acoustic signals are received incorrectly and, consequently, not processed properly so that reactions are frequently inadequate. The child is unable to tell the difference between various noises, and sounds are not imitated properly, if at all.

At times the child reacts completely unexpectedly to unpleasant noises. The child displays exceeding discomfort or covers its ears with its hands. It cries uninhibitedly.

Sound Formation with Special Attention Given to Breathing, Sucking, and Swallowing

There is a complete lack of or merely inadequate phonation without nuances. The child nearly always cries loudly; there is no modelling of sounds. Breathing, sucking, and swallowing are not coordinated; the child frequently swallows incorrectly and aspirates.

Vision and Eye Movements

Coordination is poor of the eyemuscles; strabismus is often present. Hand-eye coordination is poor. The child does not look at objects that it touches or that have been brought close to it. It does not fix its gaze on people, nor does it smile at them or even observe them. It does not follow objects or persons with its gaze after they have disappeared from direct view. A child with considerable motor disturbances is unable to follow or recognize the object, although it can see (according to tests by an eye specialist).

Routines of Daily Life

The child is not yet able to hold a cookie or piece of bread in its hand and nibble on it or eat it. Disturbances of mouth coordination, inability to recognize edibles, poor stability, and incoordination of body motoricity are reasons for such failure. The child cannot drink or eat from a spoon and sucks poorly.

Some children display a strong feeling of discomfort when being spoon-fed, because they have a disturbance in oral sensitivity. The interaction between mother and child may become very disturbed by this. Unfortunately, this is often not recognized, and furthermore, it is not understood that the child cries for this very reason.

Emotional Behavior

The child's emotinal behavior may be excessively disturbed as can be gathered from the aforementioned. Any nonrecognition and, hence, forced or developed frustration of mother and child can negatively influence the situation. The disturbed interaction between mother and child as well as between environment and child produce negative emotions within the child. These negative emotions then tend to meet with a lack of understanding by the environment which makes the situation even worse. The child does not recognize social signals, incorrectly interprets them, and consequently, processes them incorrectly. The environment reacts accordingly. Positive feedback fails to appear. The child reacts by showing its displeasure, or it hardly reacts at all.

Development

There is no stabilized development of the child. The upright position is inadequately assumed, if at all. The child is very insecure in all ways. Thus, the child appears either restless or too peaceful, which the people in its surroundings do not find disturbing at this point. The child's mental development as well as social contact appear disrupted. The environment is sometimes under the impression that the child cannot see or hear properly or that it is mentally disturbed, although this is not the case.

The signals from the child do not seem to correspond to the given situation; there is too much peace and quiet. Disturbances of the sleeping-waking rhythm may be the result. The sensory and motor integration is insufficient, and therefore, further development is substantially impeded. Socialization of the child with regard to its environment is disturbed. The environment regards the child as unpleasant and negative and rejects it, and the child, in turn, does not learn to make itself understood. The child is excessively protected and retains its regressive patterns of behavior.

8

Ninth Month

Normal

Gross Motoricity

Supine and prone positions. The child rarely takes on these positions any more. It attains the sitting position by going through the side position. Sometimes the child will first start from the prone position, then stand on all fours, enter the side position, and then come to the sitting position (Figs. **108, 109**).

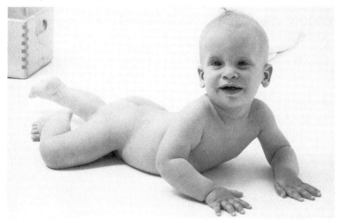

Fig. **108**

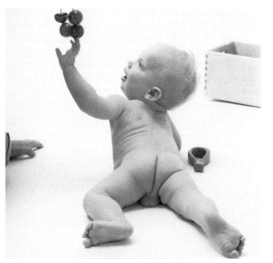

Fig. **109**

Sitting position. The child is able to sit firmly and reacts to loss of balance through counter-regulation. It can support itself in front and to the sides and has good rotation in the trunk area. The child is able to assume a symmetrical posture.

It turns around its own axis while sitting and slides forwards. Some children maintain this mode of locomotion for a considerable length of time, and therefore, start crawling rather late (Figs. **110, 111**).

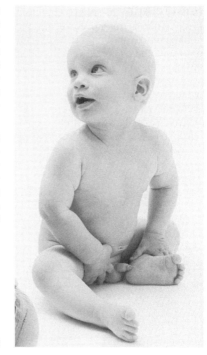

Fig. 111

Fig. **110**

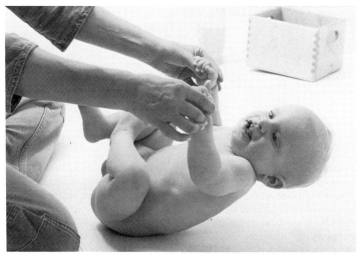

9

Pulling itself up to stand. The child pulls itself up and stands quite firmly. It bobs up and down. Balance is quite good when the child is holding onto something. It takes its first steps to the side while holding onto something (Fig. **112**).

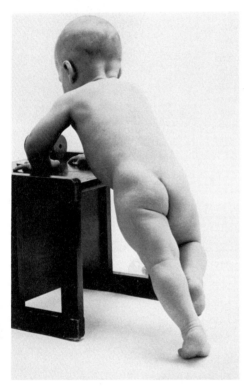

Fig. **112**

Crawling. The child is able to stand on all fours and enters this position from the sitting as well as standing position; it crawls with rotation. This way, the child is able to move about quickly, which is something it obviously enjoys. This can, of course, also prove dangerous for the child, so it must be under constant supervision. It can follow its mother or she must follow her child; this in itself is an entirely new dimension of interaction (Figs. **113, 114**).

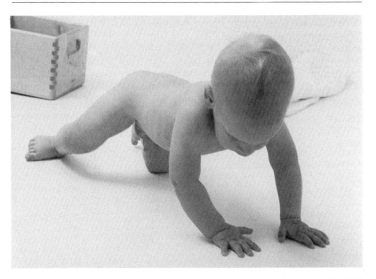

Fig. **113**

Fig. **114**

9

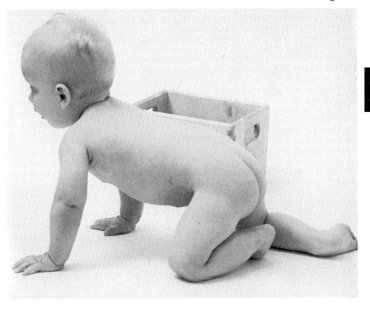

Standing. The child is able to stand while holding onto something and walks sideways along furnishings. The child can be let go of for a short period of time; however, it then falls back into the sitting position. It bobs up and down with slightly bent knees while standing. Occasional hip flexion is present, but extension is already possible. Since the child is unable to move rapidly enough when standing upright, it frequently changes from the standing position to crawling (Fig. **115**).

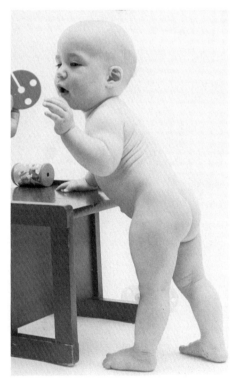

Fig. **115**

Posture and Muscle Tone

Due to the stability, tone has become regulated. Therefore, the child is able to carry out movements and retain its posture. The joints are flexible and prepared for the child to be in the upright position. There is good hip abduction.

Righting Reactions

Head positioning with respect to gravity and body image are good. If the child loses its balance, it adjusts itself through countermovements, but these are not yet stable.

Balancing Reactions

Balance in the supine, prone, and sitting positions is good. The child is capable of retaining or regaining its balance through countermovements, and it can support itself in the front as well as to the side, but not in the back. There is a good parachute and Landau reaction.

Symmetry

There is symmetrical posture. The child is capable of abandoning an asymmetrical position and reforming a symmetrical one. It is capable of working with both hands, but it distinctly prefers one.

Fine Motor Function and Adaptation

At this age, a firmly grasped toy can be released. The child grasps small objects between its thumb and bent index finger ("plier grasp" technique). It claps its hands and waves "bye-bye." It responds to the question: "How big are you?" by raising its hands to demonstrate just how big it is. There are no limitations of height yet. It is now interested in more intricate attractions such as the ticking of clocks or the telephone receiver. It points to pictures with its index finger. It attempts to hold a cup up to its mouth using both hands in order to drink from it. It removes items from its head (e.g., a scarf).

Grasping

The child grasps objects in all positions in which it can maintain balance. It reaches objects outside of its grasping range. Its hands are open, and its fingers are prepared to perform more intricate activities. The child looks at what it grasps. The child's hands come together at the midline; it plays with its hands, feet, and entire body, thus becoming acquainted with it. It touches and feels objects, thereby getting to know the difference between various materials and their pleasant and unpleasant surfaces and reacts to them by showing delight or discomfort.

It grasps small objects using the "pliers grasping" technique, i.e., with its thumb and index finger. There is good supination, and the shoulders are freely movable. There is good forward and sideways extension.

Speech and Social Contact

Speech. The child speaks in double syllables and imitates sounds it hears or produces itself. It "talks" profusely and enjoys it. It begins to whisper, i.e., to modulate its voice. There is activity at the tip of its tongue.

Social contact. Good eye contact is evident. The child smiles and has a friendly expression when it is not afraid. It understands simple questions. If one asks, "Where is Mommy?", the child will point in her direction. Strangers are observed with a skeptical expression. Any intrusion on the child's wishes is responded to by screaming. It refuses social contact if it does not wish to have any. Nonetheless, the child can be distracted. It hides behind objects and puts objects into containers and takes them out again.

Hearing and Localizing Sounds

The child listens attentively to noises and turns toward the source of the noise. It differentiates the qualities of tone. Unpleasant tones are responded to with discomfort. It hears and imitates its own noises as well as external ones.

Sound Formation with Special Attention Given to Breathing, Sucking, and Swallowing

There is good phonation with nuances, repetition, and alteration of noises. The child cries quietly and loudly, with the wish to make itself understood to its environment. It produces sounds as if telling a story. Breathing is good; sucking and swallowing are well coordinated.

Vision and Eye Movements

Good eye muscles as well as hand-eye coordination can be seen. The child looks at persons and objects. It looks at objects it has in its hands. It watches persons/objects at all levels. There is no strabismus.

Routines of Daily Life

The child begins to take a spoon into its hands and drinks from a cup that is held for it and which it can completely grasp with both hands. It eats cookies and from a spoon. Occasionally it will allow itself to be set on a potty, but there is no bowel control as yet.

Emotional Development

There is good eye contact. Social contact is good. The child only appears afraid if it actually has an obvious reason to be so. It does not like to be touched and makes its wishes distinctly known and in no uncertain terms. It chooses the people to whom it would like to relate and refuses contact with whomever it does not wish to have contact. It reacts to "no" and "yes."

The child has learned the skillful use of tactics and found weaknesses in its parents. It is curious and enjoys exploring which can, under certain circumstances, be dangerous and requires increased alertness on the parents' part. It is grateful for any help it obtains in order to reach whatever it wishes to reach as long as this help is actually in accordance with its wishes.

Development

The child has already become quite stable in the upright position. Intermediate movements improve. The child pulls itself up into the standing position and tries—still somewhat shakily—to move to the side. The surroundings are explored. The child develops mentally through its ability to alter its position with respect to gravity. It is constantly moving in order to reach something. It enjoys learning and involves its environment in this process. The mother receives signals that make it possible for her to allow her child to become more independent. She must constantly be present, because otherwise the child could hurt itself. It approaches everything and feels an urge to get to know it.

9

The child learns all the tricks necessary to make sure the people around it help it to broaden its field of activity. At this point there are many things the child prefers to do by itself, and it is up to its environment to what extent the child's gaining of independence is allowed to blossom at a normal pace.

Tenth Month

Normal

Gross Motoricity

Supine and prone positions. Some children sleep lying on their backs and some lying on their stomachs. However, this is of no significance in the examination; here the child refuses the supine position. This position is no longer assumed, and the child considers it to be unpleasant. The child immediately turns over via either side. From there it assumes the sitting position or, at times, it stand on all fours. The child begins crawling from this position (Fig. **116**).

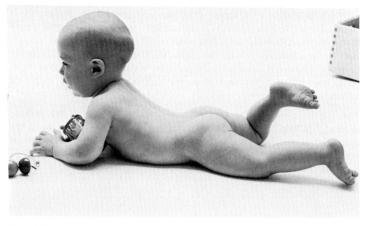

Fig. **116**

Pulling up to the sitting position. The child pulls itself up to the sitting position even without outside help (Figs. **117, 118**).

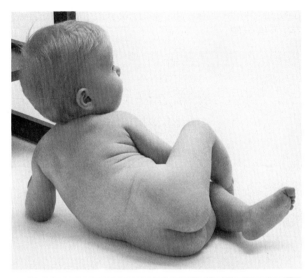

Fig. **117**

Fig. **118**

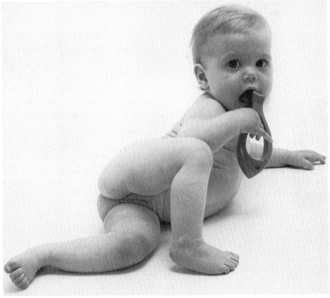

10

Sitting. The child assumes the sitting position independently and is able to balance well while sitting. It props itself up to the front, to the side, and to the back. There is good rotation. Symmetrical posture is possible. While sitting, the child can slide forward and around its own axis (Fig. **119**).

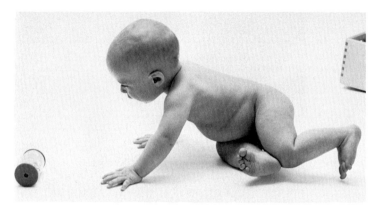

Fig. **119**

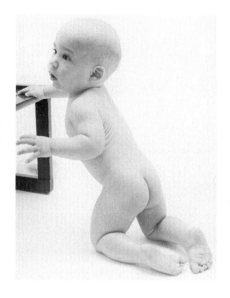

Pulling itself up to a standing position. The child uses objects to pull itself up, although it is occasionally able to stand up without this help. The child is able to stand quite firmly when holding onto something and takes sidesteps along objects (Fig. **120**).

Fig. **120**

Crawling. The child is able to crawl quickly and with good rotation. It stands on all fours coming out of both the sitting and standing position. This mode of locomotion is carefully monitored by the child's environment, because the child continuously gets itself into dangerous situations in order to grasp and comprehend everything it sees (Figs. **121, 122**).

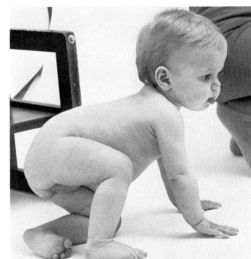

Fig. **121**

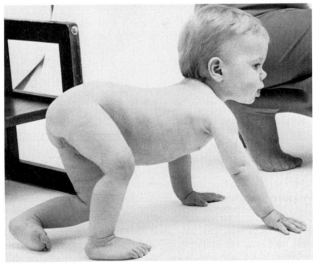

Fig. **122**

Standing. Occasionally it lets go, but it is not yet able to take steps. It mainly walks alongside pieces of furniture by taking sidesteps. The child displays considerable stability. It can sit down from this position. The intermediate stages of movements are quite good. Frequently the child goes from the standing to the crawling position (Fig. **123**).

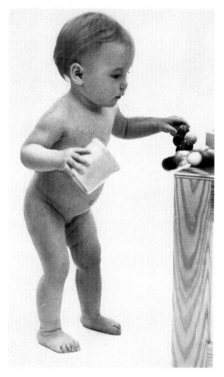

Fig. **123**

Posture and Muscle Tone

Good tone regulation which corresponds to the tension required for motor function is evident. Those joints which work against gravity are well prepared for standing upright and walking. Intermediate movements depend on a well-regulated tone. There is good hip abduction.

Righting Reactions

There are good righting reactions with respect to space.

Balancing Reactions

There is good balancing in the supine, prone, and sitting positions, but not while standing as yet. Good reactions are shown when balance is lost. The child can prop itself up well.

Symmetry

Symmetrical posture is consistently possible. The child assumes symmetrical posture directly from an asymmetrical one. It works with both hands but shows an obvious preference for one.

Fine Motor Function and Adaptation

The child passes toys around and sometimes releases one. It throws toys down and expects the adult to pick them up and start playing the game all over again. The child grasps small objects with its thumb and index finger ("pliers grasping" technique).

The child takes objects out of a container and puts them back. It does not yet find objects that have been hidden right before its eyes. It is interested in smaller attractions such as the ticking of a clock. It enjoys playing with the telephone but only by listening. It plays with dice and similar objects with considerable concentration. It drinks from a cup and even holds it with both hands if the cup is handed to it.

Grasping

The child reaches for objects from any position in which it is able to retain balance. It reaches objects that are outside of its actual grasping range. Its hands are open, and its fingers are prepared for more intricate activities.

10

The child looks at whatever it grasps. Its hands come together at the midline. The child plays with its hands, feet, and entire body, thus getting to know its body better. It touches and feels objects and becomes acquainted with various materials as well as with the difference between pleasant and unpleasant surfaces, to which it responds with pleasure or discomfort.

The child grasps small objects by using its thumb and bent index finger ("pliers grasping" technique). There is good supination with freely movable shoulders. The child passes objects from one hand to the other (hand-to-hand coordination). There is good forward extension as well as sideways and backwards movements.

Speech and Social Contact

Speech. The child speaks double syllables chainwise. "Mommy" and "Daddy" are spoken without being properly addressed. It reacts when hearing its name and to demands such as "give me". It imitates sounds that it makes itself or hears and likes to "talk". It modulates its voice to be loud or soft and sometimes it whispers. It plays with its tongue and saliva in order to produce sounds.

Social contact. The child begins to understand when it is being reprimanded or praised. It does as the mother wishes and what it will be praised for doing. If it wishes to do something for which it has been reprimanded, it uses tricks. The child responds to demands with the means it has at this age, e.g., looks at the person with whom it is communicating at the time. Strangers are looked at with skepticism, but the child is willing to take up contact. It either laughs out loud or smiles. Nonetheless, the child will refuse to take up contact if it feels uncomfortable doing so or does not wish to. Pleasure and discomfort are made known. With understanding, it is possible to distract the child.

The child plays hide-and-seek and begins to play with others instead of merely alongside them.

Hearing and Localizing Sounds

The child becomes attentive when it hears noises and turns toward their sources. It differentiates between the qualities of noises. It responds to unpleasant noises with discomfort. It hears its own sounds as well as external noises and imitates them.

Sound Formation with Special Attention Given to Breathing, Sucking, and Swallowing

Good phonation with nuances, repetition, and alteration of noises is evident. The child cries softly or loudly, desiring to make itself understood to its environment. Breathing is good; sucking and swallowing are well coordinated.

Vision and Eye Movements

Eye-muscle and hand-eye coordination are good. It looks at persons and objects. It looks at objects it has in its hands. It watches them at all levels. There is no strabismus.

Routines of Daily Life

The child takes the spoon into its hand with the intention of eating by itself, but it must still be fed. It drinks from a cup that is held toward it and grasps it with both hands. It then drinks from the cup by itself; it eats cookies. Occasionally it will allow itself to be set on the potty, but it has as yet no bladder control.

Emotional Behavior

Good eye contact and good social contact are noted. The child only seems afraid if it has an obvious reason. It does not like to be touched and distinctly expresses its desires. It choses the people to whom it wishes to relate and refuses contact with the remainder. It reacts to the words "no" and "yes." It has already learned about the benefits of skillful tactics and has discovered some weak points in its parents.

The child is curious and enjoys exploring its environment, which can, in some cases, be dangerous and requires increased alertness from the parents. The child is grateful for any help it can get so long as this help caters to its wishes.

Development

This is the age of transition between the horizontal and—still unstable—vertical position. Intermediate movements improve. The child pulls itself up into a standing position and tries to let go and stand by itself. It moves along the furnishings and crawls. At this age, it begins to worry the people around it. The child cannot be left alone any more, because it touches everything and pulls it down.

However, this is the child's way of exploring its environment. The people that are part of its environment are constantly teaching it things, because the child demands this. The child learns very rapidly at this age. The preparations for walking upright and for speech have already been completed. Now the child starts to move about in this upright position and to use the speech it has learned. It listens and produces many sounds itself. It becomes more and more independent, which it likes. The child's contacts to its environment become more differentiated, and it chooses and reacts with emotion. This has a signal effect on the child's environment.

10

Twelfth Month

Normal

Gross Motoricity

Supine and prone positions. The child rests in these positions only when sleeping and not during its waking hours. The supine position is uncomfortable for the child. It turns over via both sides. It achieves the sitting position by going through the sideways sitting position. It stands on all fours in order to crawl.

Pulling itself up to a sitting position. The child pulls itself up to a sitting position but would be able to enter this position even without pulling by doing a half turn.

Sitting. The child is able to sit by itself and displays good balance and is capable of propping itself up on all sides. There is good lengthwise sitting posture displaying good hip flexion and an extended back. The legs are outwardly rotated. There is good rotation and symmetrical posture (Fig. **124**).

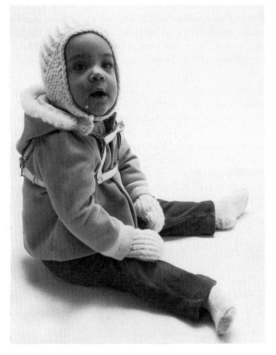

Fig. **124**

Pulling itself up into the standing position. The child is capable of pulling itself up into the standing position, but sometimes it stands up without any outside support or by way of the "bear" standing position. Some children are already able to move themselves forward, departing from the standing position and taking only a few steps. Balance is not yet very stable. The child moves along furniture. It does so rather quickly. It likes to change to the crawling position and crawls rapidly (Fig. **125**).

Fig. **125**

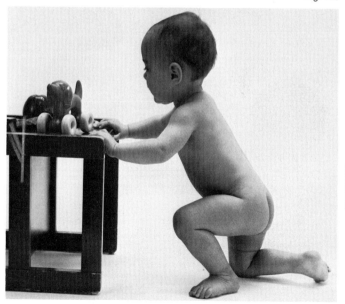

12

Crawling. The child crawls while displaying rotation and balance. At this time, it still prefers the quicker mode of locomotion. From this position it enters the sitting and standing positions. This mode of locomotion is dangerous, and the persons around the child must keep a watchful eye on it so that it does not get hurt (Figs. **126, 127**).

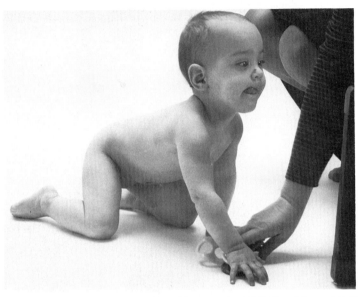

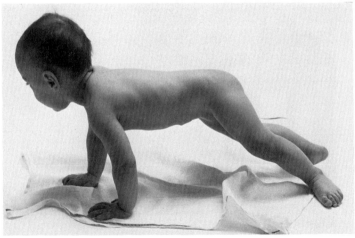

Standing and Walking. The child can stand on its own without holding on to anything. At this time, the child often does not yet display balance and is frequently unable to leave the position in which it stands. Sometimes it takes a few uncertain steps with its legs apart. When moving to sit down, the child already displays good intermediate stages of steps (Fig. **128**).

◀ Fig. **126**

◀ Fig. **127**

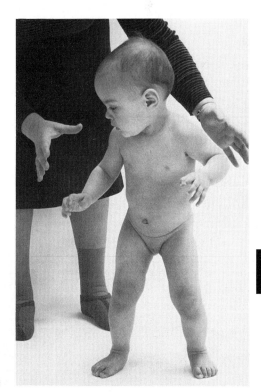

Fig. **128**

Posture and Muscle Tone

The tone is regulated in such a way that the child is able to function well despite the lack of balance. The joints which work against gravity are well prepared for the upright position. The intermediate stages of movements are quite good. Hip abduction is good.

Righting Reactions

There are good righting reactions with respect to space (Figs. **129, 130**).

Figs. **129, 130**

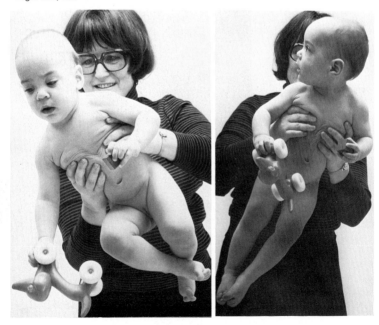

Balancing Reactions

There is good balance in the supine, prone, and sitting positions as well as when crawling. The child is still somewhat insecure when standing but has good reactions on loss of balance; there is good propping up on its arms (Fig. **131**).

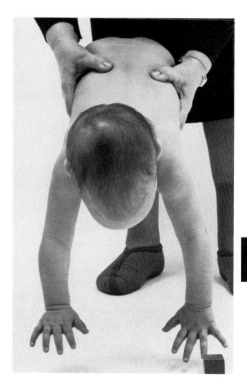

Fig. **131**

Fine Motor Function and Adaptation

The child takes toys out of a toybox and puts them back in again. It passes toys on to others, thereby releasing them, finds hidden toys, and puts small objects through narrow openings, e.g., through a bottleneck. It pulls toys toward itself or along behind it.

It takes things out of a container and puts them back again. A coin is picked up with the thumb and index finger using the "pliers grasping" technique. Even tiny crumbs are picked up very skillfully. It drinks from a cup by itself when the cup is put into its hands.

It enjoys playing with a telephone, listens to it intensively, and is interested in more sophisticated stimuli such as the ticking of a watch.

The child concentrates when it plays. It sets dice one on top of the other. It bangs two dice together.

Grasping

The child grasps for objects from all positions in which it can maintain balance. It can also reach objects outside of its range. Its hands are open, and its fingers are ready to perform finer activities.

The child looks at whatever it grasps. Its hands join at the midline, and it plays with its hands, feet, and entire body. It touches and feels objects and becomes acquainted with materials and learns to tell the difference between pleasant and unpleasant surfaces, to which it reacts by demonstrating pleasure or discomfort.

It grasps small objects with its thumb and curved index finger using the "pliers grasping" technique. There is good supination with freely moveable shoulders and exchange of objects from one hand to the other by crossing at the midline (hand-to-hand coordination).

There is good forward arm extension as well as to the side and backwards.

Speech and Social Contact

Speech. The child says 1–3 words that have a meaning such as "ham-ham", "wow-wow", "ga-ga". The words "Papa" and "Mama" are directed towards those persons. It reacts to its name as well as to demands such as "give me ..." and, for a short period, to orders such as "no" and "yes." It imitates sounds that it hears or produces itself. It loves to "talk" and does so a lot. It modulates its voice to be loud and soft; it sometimes whispers. It plays with its tongue and saliva in order to produce noises. It already has good language understanding.

Social contact. It understands when it is being reprimanded or praised. It does whatever the mother wishes in order to please her when she praises it. Nevertheless, whenever it has wishes of its own, it already uses tricks to achieve what it wants. It notices quite well when it irritates the persons around it. It is well able to use its position as a helpless being. It reacts to demands by using the means that are at a child's disposal at this age, such as a long glance, etc. Unfamiliar persons are regarded skeptically, but the child is prepared to take up contact. It laughs out loud or smiles. However, it refuses contact if it is not in the mood or it does not feel comfortable doing so. Pleasure and discomfort are made known. The child can be distracted; however, one must adapt to its needs. It makes its desires known without screaming. It plays with other people (rolling a ball back and forth). It likes to play hide-and-seek and enjoys looking in a mirror where it is able to recognize itself as well as others. Some children are already able to eat with a spoon by themselves. The child plays with others and not merely beside them.

Hearing and Localizing Sounds

The child listens attentively when it hears noises and turns toward their sources. It differentiates various qualities of noise. Unpleasant noises are responded to with discomfort. It hears its own sounds and imitates them as well as outside noises. The child speaks its first words.

Routines of Daily Life

The child takes the spoon into its hands but must still be fed. It drinks from a cup that is held towards it and emcompasses the cup with both hands. It drinks from the cup by itself. It eats bread and cookies.

The child allows itself to be placed on the potty occasionally. The development of the child's feeling for cleanliness depends upon guidance by the parents. There is initial bladder control.

Emotional Behavior

There is good eye contact and social contact. The child only appears frightened if it actually has a reason to be. It does not like to be touched and makes its needs and wishes known distinctly. It chooses the persons to whom it wishes to relate and refuses contact with others. It has learned to use skillful tactics as well as to discover its parents' weak spots. It is curious and enjoys exploring its surroundings, which can be somewhat dangerous for the child and requires the parents to be very watchful. The child is grateful for any help that is suited to achieve satisfaction of its needs.

12

Development

The child has become more stable in the upright position, although not yet completely so. The intermediate movements have continued to improve. The child is able to pull itself up to the standing position and take some steps with its legs apart, although somewhat unsteadily.

The child still crawls in order to get about but attempts to move in the upright position more frequently. One cannot leave the child alone, because it touches everything and pulls it down. This is the child's way of getting to know its surroundings. The people around the child are constantly teaching it things as it demands. At this age, the child learns many things very rapidly. Preparations for speaking have taken place. It now begins to speak. It becomes increasingly more independent, which it finds pleasing. Contact with the environment becomes more differentiated. It picks and chooses and reacts with emotions. These emotions have a signal effect on its environment.

Fifteenth Month

Normal

Gross Motoricity

Supine and prone positions. These are not maintained as positions. The child turns via both sides to the sideways sitting position and then to the sitting position, or it goes from standing on all fours or the "bearlike" standing position to crawling and walking. In most cases it can walk without extra support but still does so with its legs apart.

Sitting. The child sits with very good balance and can prop itself up for support on all sides. There is good lengthwise sitting with bent hips and extended back. The legs are outwardly rotated. There is good rotation and symmetrical posture (Fig. **132**).

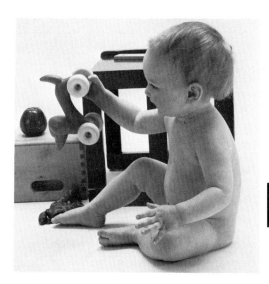

Fig. **132**

15

Crawling. Crawling is no longer the child's mode of locomotion, but it can still be used. It is coordinated (Fig. **133**).

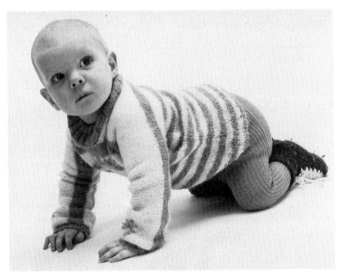

Fig. **133**

Standing. The child stands up and is also able to enter another position from the standing position. It is capable of shifting its weight and is readily able to adapt to alterations in position (Figs. **134, 135**).

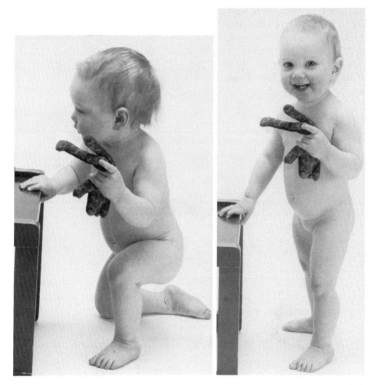

Fig. **134**   Fig. **135**

15

Walking. The child is able to walk on its own; its sense of balance is not yet completely developed. Occasionally it walks with its legs apart. Some 75% of all children are able to walk at this age. While it walks, the child is able to hold an object in its hands (both hands) or to stretch its arms out in order to grasp something. Sometimes the legs are still inwardly rotated, and hence the feet are pointed toward the inside. The child may even trip over its own feet. The child's feet lie flat on the underlying surface, showing no arch; however, during the examination it may actually be visible. The joints are easily moveable.

Posture and Muscle Tone

Normal postural and muscle tone are evident.

Righting Reactions

There are good righting reactions in all positions (Fig. **136**).

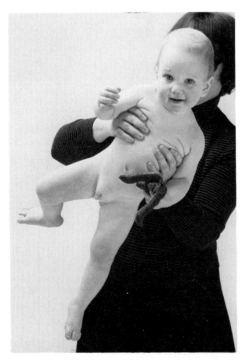

Fig. **136**

Balancing Reactions

There is good balance when lying and sitting; balance is already quite good when standing and walking as well. However, the child's balance when walking is still unstable. There is good propping up.

Fine Motor Function and Adaptation

Due to the child's ability to walk, it approaches objects and grasps them. It imitates its mother and will perform certain small duties that are asked of it. It eats with a spoon by itself but still spills quite a lot. It can take off some pieces of clothing. It scribbles if given a pencil. It builds a tower with two blocks. It takes toys out of a box and puts them back in. It pulls toys along behind it or toward itself. It arranges objects but does not categorize them yet. It throws them all together. Tiny crumbs or threads are picked up skillfully. It drinks from a cup. The child plays with considerable concentration and arranges blocks.

Grasping

The child grasps objects from any position in which it has good balance. It grasps objects that are out of its reach. Its hands are open and in supination, and its fingers are freely moveable and extended, thus prepared for more intricate activities. Good hand-eye and hand-hand coordination is noted. The hands meet at the midline. The child is able to pick up smaller objects or turn the pages of a book quite skillfully by using its thumb and index finger ("pliers grasping" technique); however, this movement is occasionally somewhat exaggerated. The shoulders are easily moveable, and the arms can be extended with ease.

The child touches things with considerable sensitivity and distinguishes between various materials and surfaces. It shows feelings of pleasure and discomfort accordingly.

Speech and Social Contact

Speech. The child says the words "Mommy" and "Daddy," directing these terms correctly, and sometimes speaks more words. There is good understanding of language. If prompted to do so, the child will pass objects that it has taken into a person's hands. It reacts when its name is called as well as to the words "yes" and "no". It says words that make sense such as "ham-ham," "ga-ga," or "bow-bow". It imitates noises, e.g., motor noises. It attempts to tell "stories" and even changes tone. It whispers.

Social contact. The child understands quite well what adults wish it to do or when it is being praised or reprimanded. It makes its own wishes known and carries them through, if need be by using tricks. It reacts to demands placed on it and fulfills them. The child is proud if it successfully accomplishes a task. It takes up contact on its own initiative but refuses contact if it dislikes the object/person. It laughs and cries and makes pleasure and discomfort known. The child allows itself to become distracted if one gives in to its needs.

It plays "hide-and-seek" with other children. It is willing to play real games with adults. It eats with others when sitting properly at the table. It takes the spoon and eats with hardly any mess at all.

Hearing and Localizing Sounds

The ability to hear and localize noises is good.

Routines of Daily Life

The child eats with a spoon and drinks from a cup. It eats bread by itself but makes quite a mess. It allows itself to be put on a potty and understands that it is supposed to learn to control its bladder this way. Since this learning process is strongly linked to psychological factors such as the mother-child relationship, details pertaining to the child's development of bowel control can be made only with certain reservations.

Emotional Behavior

The child's emotional behavior is well balanced.

Development

The child is still not quite stable when in the upright position, but it is capable of moving around well enough to allow it to examine its surroundings. Intermediate stages of movements have improved substantially. If the child is moving about by itself, it is capable of squatting to pick up an object from the floor.

One cannot leave the child alone any more; it touches and tries out everything. Every day it learns something new, and it knows its environment. Speech development is a priority at this age, and through this a new dimension opens for the child.

Visual, acoustic, and tactile-kinesthetic perception display integrational tendencies (Figs. **137–142**).

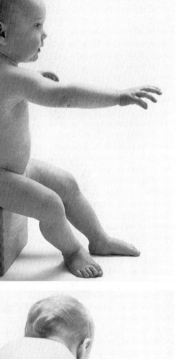

Fig. **137**

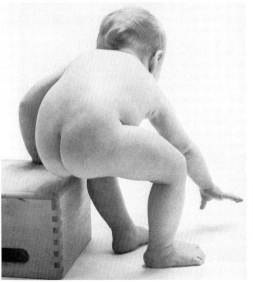

Fig. **138**

15

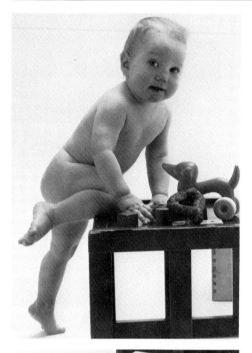

Fig. **139**

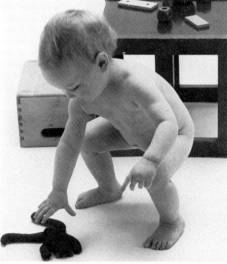

Fig. **140**

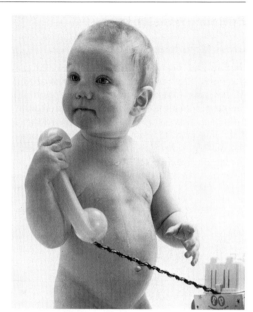

Fig. **141**

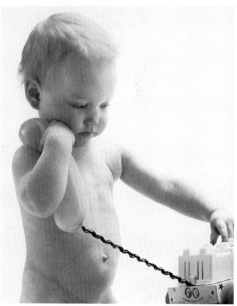

Fig. **142**

Deviating Development

Gross Motoricity

Supine and prone positions. If the child remains in either of these positions, there is a distinct persistence of tonic postural patterns such as excessive extension in the supine position and excessive flexion in the prone position. The remaining pattern is in accordance with preference, e.g., excessive flexor or extensor tone. Posture is asymmetrical. The child is either completely unable to turn over from both sides, or this task is only possible with great difficulties. There is a poor or inadequate ability to lift its head. This is sometimes better in one position than in another. The abdominal wall is floppy (Figs. **143**, **144**).

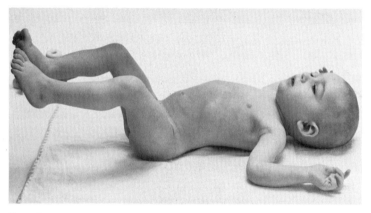

Fig. **143**

Fig. **144**

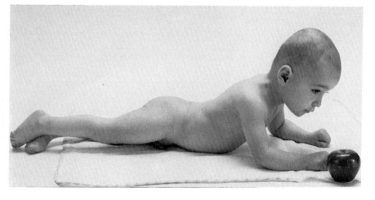

Sitting. It takes great effort on the child's behalf to enter the sitting position if it is able to do so at all. If the child is placed in the sitting position, it is unstable and does not prop itself up optimally on both sides; occasionally it does so towards the front as a way of keeping itself straight. When sitting lengthwise, the child displays inhibited hip flexion as well as a hunched back as a mode of compensation. In cases of atony, a child may display an especially straight back which is caused by exaggerated tone. Occasionally one notes the hunched back without inhibited hip flexion. The legs display excessive outward or inward rotation with adduction. There is poor rotation; asymmetrical posture is seen frequently (Fig. **145**).

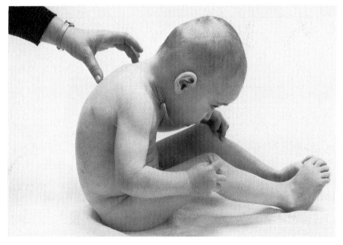

Fig. **145**

15

Crawling. The child is not capable of crawling since it is too floppy. Should it crawl at all, it does so with poor rotation. The arms can be moved better than the legs, especially in diparetic children. In less severe cases of quadruplegia, the ATNR is occasionally still present, making coordinated crawling nearly impossible. The same holds true for a persistent STNR or TLR (Fig. **146**).

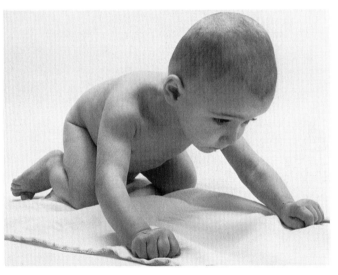

Fig. **146**

Standing. From time to time and with a great amount of effort, the child is able to use objects to pull itself up. In floppy/atonic children one notes considerable contraction with recurvature of the knees. There is aggravation of intermediate stages of movements. The body weight cannot be shifted properly, which leads to disturbances of balance. The ability to stand without holding onto something is sometimes possible, but the child is quite unsteady (Fig. **147**).

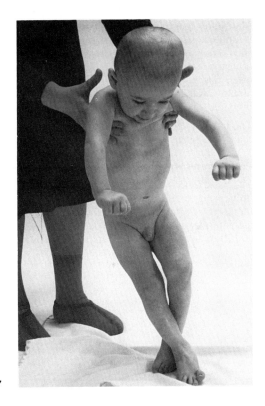

Fig. **147**

15

Walking. It is not possible for an abnormally developed child to walk as it cannot maintain balance when it is in an upright position. Persistent tonic posture patterns prevent this in many cases. Steady walking is not possible until the child has a sense of balance when standing.

Some children hold themselves in an upright position although their tone is not properly regulated. They are very uncoordinated and fall down easily, but nevertheless they walk despite the fact that they fall forward and must catch something to hold them.

The child's feet frequently display considerable inward rotation, which is understandable due to inadequate hip rotation. Such symptoms should only be considered a case of delayed development if the child is otherwise symmetrical and displays no alterations of tone. The child often has both talipes planus and pes valgus, although the arch is already well formed. The ankle joint does not appear well enough prepared for the upright position.

The hips also appear to be widely abductable and unstable. The joints that work against gravity are floppy.

Posture and Muscle Tone

The basic tone is either hypertonic, hypotonic, or alternating, thereby influencing stability when standing upright. There is altered mobility of the joints. Posture and the maintenance thereof are impaired. Intermediate movements are not adequately possible. Hip abduction and adduction are altered. Persistent tonic postural patterns influence tone distribution in the muscular system, thereby strengthening tone alterations.

Righting Reactions

Righting reactions are, for the most part, inadequate and are not sufficient for body positioning with respect to space. Due to a lack of stability, head control is poor. This becomes especially visible when the child attempts to pull itself up from the supine to the upright position. Upon loss of balance, the child's head does not respond sufficiently, and therefore, it loses its balance more rapidly (Fig. **148**).

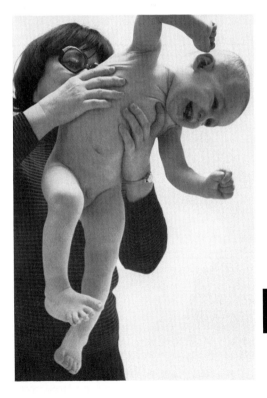

Fig. **148**

Balancing Reactions

The child does not display adequate balance in any position. Occasionally, balance is quite good in the prone and supine positions, but this ceases in all upright positions. If the child lacks balance when sitting or crawling, this will also be the case when standing or walking. Regulation as well as counter-regulation upon loss of balance are poor. Inadequate balance increases the child's fear considerably and makes it psychologically insecure, which results in hesitant and fearful behavior. As soon as the child notices that it will be helped if it loses its balance, it becomes more secure. However, the child can rely too heavily on this help and become slightly scared when it fails. Sometimes when the child falls, it is unable to give itself proper support and falls with a complete lack of regulation. This lack of balance is a considerable burden to the mother-child relationship, because the child's poor and extremely fearful reactions bring forth a feeling of failure in the mother (Fig. **149**).

Fig. **149**

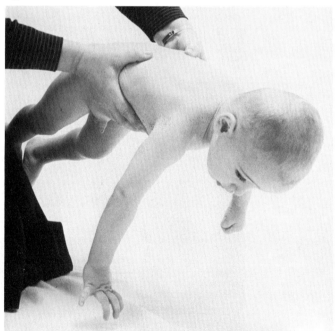

Symmetry

Positions are assumed asymmetrically and cannot become symmetrical. The child consistently prefers one side, while the other is not even noticed. Either only the upper or only the lower extremities are affected. The affected side is hardly looked at and not used for motor activities. If one observes very precisely, one will notice that the side that is not as severely affected also displays some conspicuous signs but that these signs are considerably weaker.

Fine Motor Function and Adaptation

Due to the child's lack of movement, it is dependent on the position it has assumed. If the child is stabilized, it grasps for objects in a very uncoordinated manner. Occasionally, it grasps using only one hand while the other acts as a helping hand. The hand displays associated reactions that become more pronounced when in action. The hand sometimes forms a fist and goes into pronation. The arm bends considerably, with shoulder retraction. This hand is not often looked at. Hand-eye coordination may be poor. When grasping, the child's movement is very imprecise, even if it looks at the object. If the child is not satisfied with its movement, it gives up. Objects outside of the child's range can only be reached if the child's mobility is sufficient. Activities at the midline, such as hand clapping, are frequently not possible. It is frequently impossible for the child to release an object it is holding due to persistence of the grasping reflex. The child does not bother to keep watching falling objects but rather loses interest in them quickly. The child glances around anxiously, which makes focusing on objects difficult. It appears to lack concentration since it loses eye contact with both objects and persons very quickly. The child appears to have autistic characteristics. Persons that are around the child a lot often think it is mentally handicapped.

Noises and visual stimuli are incorrectly interpreted by the child and cause it to become frightened. The child's reactions are inadequate. The child is unable to adjust to changes quickly enough, which leads to its having a large number of failures. The child signals discomfort, or it resigns and becomes stubborn and sluggish.

Grasping

Well-directed grasping only becomes possible if the child is stabilized (sometimes rather difficult when dealing with a floppy child). Slowly performed movements are displayed by children with a high basic tone.

15

The inadequacy of the righting and balancing reactions generates discomfort in the child since it is unable to move about freely. Instead, it is constantly made to feel insecure. The child does experience tactile sensations; however, since the signals are incorrect, it is not capable of processing them.

The child's poor sense of space as well as false tactile information make it feel uncomfortable and insecure. Its reactions towards the environment are disturbed. It does not possess enough control when grasping; hence, the grasp is either too weak or too strong. This is another reason why materials are often percieved incorrectly, and differentiation is almost impossible.

If the child is unable to receive signals properly, the reactions cannot be adapted to the given situation. Interaction with the environment becomes full of misunderstanding and, hence, confusing. The child signals discomfort, which is frequently misinterpreted by its environment. Small objects cannot be grasped, and the child misses the objects, thus frequently experiencing failure. Hand-eye coordination is inadequate, meaning that the child is unable to look correctly at persons or objects. Three-dimensional experiences, such as stereoscopic vision, cannot develop. Objects do not stand out against their backgrounds properly. Dysgnosia and, later, dyspraxia may arise.

Speech and Social Contact

Speech. If the child has disturbances in mouth coordination, its articulation will be disturbed (dysarthria). Expressive speech is impaired. Speech behavior may be disturbed due to a receptive dysphasia; however, it is usually quite good, which is recognizable in the child's behavior.

At this age, the child begins to point at parts of its body that have been pointed out to it and named. From an understanding point of view, the child is usually capable of bringing objects it is asked to bring. It reacts to its name if it is able to hear. If it does not do this, it is able to hear but does not relate the sounds it hears to itself (hearing test by a doctor is necessary). It does not understand the words "yes" and "no" because it is unable to interpret these expressions even though it hears them. Not only can speech development at this time be considered disturbed, since the preliminary steps are lacking, but also the inability to imitate sounds. In most cases, a hearing disturbance exists if a child of this age does not imitate sounds; however, it could also be due to disturbed processing.

Furthermore, acoustic perception may be disturbed. This means that the noises are incorrectly received at a central point and, hence, are incorrectly expressed. Some of these sounds generate discomfort in the child, and the child makes this known.

Social contact. The child's contact with its environment may be considerably disturbed; nonetheless, the causes—which are often quite diverse—must be found.

Poor eye fixation and poor processing of acoustic signals are enough to cause disturbances in the interaction between the child and its environment. These children sometimes appear blind or deaf. If, in addition, the child shows a tactile-kinesthetic disturbance, it will appear mentally handicapped. Autistic characteristics are not rare in such cases. Information about the early part of the child's infancy can be very helpful, e.g., discomfort at first spoon-feeding (disturbance of mouth sensitivity), shrill, inadequate crying in response to noises and visual impressions, poor development of head control, and considerable instability in the upright position.

Excessive anxiety when confronted with unfamiliar persons—a trait which is no longer typical at this age—as well as excessive friendliness toward unfamiliar persons or uncontrolled smiling should give cause for increased observation of the child.

Some mothers are very sensitive in this respect and are able to describe such behavior in great detail. One should listen attentively when the mother talks about this.

Hearing and Localizing Sounds

The child does not immediately turn toward the source of noise as it either does not recognize or does not localize the noise. The child should undergo hearing tests by a specialist in order to ensure that it is really able to hear correctly. Acoustic signals are either incorrectly received and thus incorrectly processed, or they are correctly received but not recognized correctly. The reactions seem inadequate.

Various noises are not differentiated, hence they cannot—if at all—be properly imitated.

The child reacts in an unexpected manner to some noises that do not sound unpleasant to most people. The child displays discomfort, places its hands over its ears, and cries without inhibition.

Sound Formation with Special Attention Given to Breathing, Sucking, and Swallowing

There is poor phonation without nuances. The sounds are not modulated. The child either cries excessively or hardly makes any noise at all. Breathing, sucking, and swallowing are sometimes not very well coordinated. The child frequently swallows incorrectly or aspirates.

Vision and Eye Movements

There is poor coordination of eyemuscles and strabismus. Hand-eye coordination is not good; the child does not look at objects that it touches or that are brought close to it. At this age, disturbances in visual perception already become noticeable, which make the child quite irritated. Persons are not focused upon or smiled at or even looked at adequately. The child does not follow objects or persons with its gaze after they have gone out of its range of view. The child is unable to follow objects with its eyes, or it does not recognize objects although it sees them (vision should also be tested by a specialist).

Routines of Daily Life

In some cases, the child does not yet eat by itself, because the mother prefers to feed it and has not yet taught it to become more independent. The question here is whether the child would be capable of doing certain things if it were allowed to do so (some spilling permitted). The child is frequently unable to chew since its oral coordination is poor. Hypersensitivity in the mouth area prevents the child from eating, for example, with a spoon. If the child is forced to do so, the interaction between mother and child may become considerably disturbed. A child's eating by itself is also dependent upon motor stability. Poor motor coordination keeps the child from drinking from a mug or cup.

Poor stability also prevents development of bladder control, whenever the attempt is made to train the child on a potty. If this is done too early, severe disturbances in bladder control may be the result. Learning disturbances hamper this development since bladder control requires not only a certain amount of maturity but also a substantial ability to learn.

Emotional Behavior

After what has just been said, it is not surprising that emotional disturbances also occur. The inability to recognize disturbances often leads to demands being enforced, which, in turn, increase the child's and the mother's frustration and negatively influences their behavior. This disturbed interaction between mother and child as well as between the environment and the child generates negative emotions in the child. These generally meet with a lack of understanding from the people around it, which makes the situation even worse. Social signals are not properly recognized and thus interpreted and processed falsely. The child's environment reacts accordingly. Positive feedback does not occur. The child either reacts by showing its discomfort, or it hardly reacts at all. The latter is frequently misinterpreted as the child acting "well behaved."

Development

In contrast to a healthy child, this type of child has not yet attained stability in the upright position. The child's lack of experience with its environment, which is also due to this, becomes obvious through its behavior. It is either too quiet or too fidgety and loud. At this time, it is already appropriate to speak of these children as hyperkinetic. Basically, all difficulties that the older child has are already visible at this age, but they are more readily tolerated by the environment now than later. The child itself attempts to direct these conspicuous signs but fails to do so, making the situation even worse. It is almost impossible to leave such a fidgety child alone without it starting to cry. It cries to protest a lack of stimulation from outside, as it uses its environment (as does a healthy child) to create experiences. All of the child's responses resemble over-responses.

Speech and mental development do not yet seem to be as conspicuous at this age as they do some months later; however, they must be recognized now in order to prevent further faulty developments. Early diagnosis appears very difficult, especially since there is a variation in normal development. Defective interaction between the child and its environment cannot be recognized without a substantial observation period.

The information which has been gathered up to now pertaining to this age period is rather limited.

15

Eighteenth Month

Normal

Gross Motoricity

The child displays good balance in all positions. It can lie on its back symmetrically, turn to the prone position via both sides, as well as turn to support itself on all fours and then into the sitting position. There is good head and trunk control as well as good rotation. Hip flexion when sitting and hip extension when standing are good.

When walking, the child still has physiological pes valgoplanus despite good plantar arching being felt. The legs are sometimes still slightly inwardly rotated and the rotation of the hips is inadequate.

There is good mobility of the joints. There are still associated movements. The child is capable of carrying an object in each hand when walking. It can stoop down, thereby displaying good intermediate stages of movements, in order to pick up an object from the floor. It

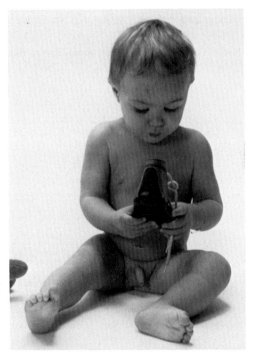

Fig. **150**

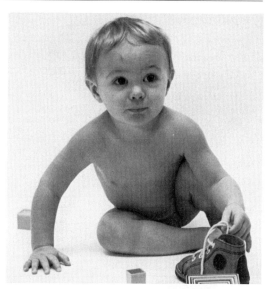

Fig. **151**

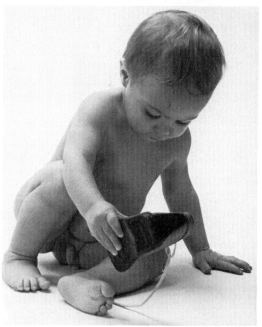

Fig. **152**

18

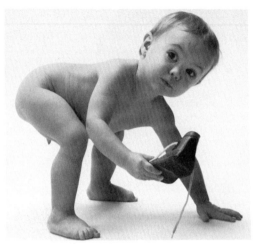

Figs. **153–155**

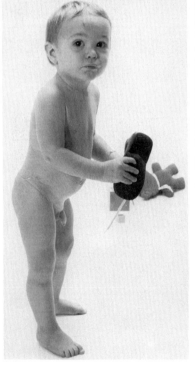

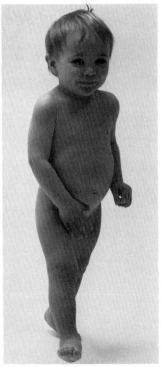

can walk backwards and play "soccer." From a standing position, the child is able to throw a ball in an overhand manner. When held by the hand, the child can climb stairs. It is already able to stop itself with ease when walking (Figs. **150–155**).

Balancing Reactions

There is good balance in all positions. Stability is already quite substantial. There is good propping up on the hands. Balance is not yet adequate when standing, hopping on one leg, or carrying out the straight-line walking test. However, the child practices constantly while playing and gets into situations that require optimal adaptation (Fig. **156**).

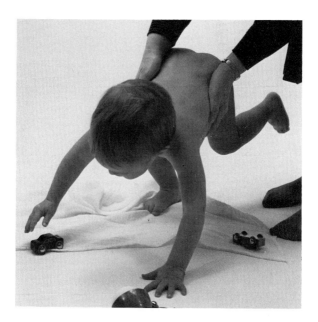

Fig. **156**

For this reason, difficult situations arise from time to time which require the attention of an adult, but constant intervention is no longer necessary. The child can throw a ball without falling.

18

Fine Motor Function and Adaptation

The child grasps objects and carries them around. It imitates household chores and helps if it is asked to do simple tasks. It eats with a spoon by itself but still grasps the spoon in pronation.

It takes off clothing, drinks from a cup by itself, and scribbles if given a pencil. It will build a tower out of four blocks, put toys into a toybox, and take them back out again. It is able to remember where objects are hidden if they are put into the toybox while the child is watching.

The child organizes objects and even tries to categorize them. It unpacks wrapped objects and throws things away. It touches and differentiates between various materials and surfaces. It uses its index finger alone. It clears things out and puts things away. It plays with great concentration and fantasy (Figs. **157, 158**).

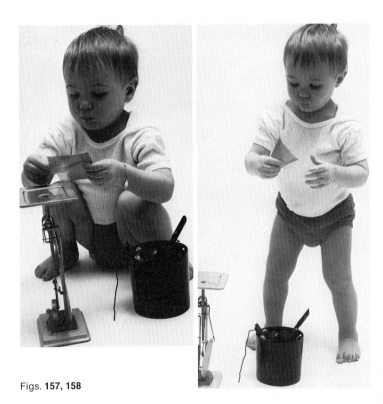

Figs. **157, 158**

Grasping

The child grasps objects from all positions. It reaches objects that are outside of its range. Its hands are open and supinated, but grasping, e.g., of a pencil, still occasionally takes place in pronation. Its fingers can be intricately manipulated. There is good hand-eye and hand-hand coordination. The hands meet at the midline. The child grasps fine objects with its thumb and bent index finger ("pliers-grasping" position). The child can turn the page of a book. It becomes continuously more dexterous in doing so.

The shoulders are moveable at all levels, and the arms can be extended. When examining adiadochokinesia, strong associated movements of one side and uncoordination due to the same movement originating at the shoulder can still be noted. The hands turn well and symmetrically. The child touches objects with a great amount of sensitivity and differentiates between various materials and surfaces which the mother should name.

Speech and Social Contact

Speech. The child says "Mommy" and "Daddy" as well as a few other words. It is sometimes able to speak two words which are related in meaning, one after the other. There is good understanding of speech. It places objects that it has picked up into its hand if asked to do so. It reacts to its name and understands the words "yes" and "no" as well as the meaning of praise and reprimand. It imitates its own sounds as well as external noises such as motor noises and animal noises, etc.

Social contact. It fully participates in family life. It can sit at the table at mealtime and eat cut-up food with a spoon by itself. It drinks from a cup.

It understands what is asked of it and does as it is told. It reacts to praise and reprimand by showing pleasure or discomfort. It is quite good at getting its way, sometimes even doing so with tricks. It is proud when it succeeds in fulfilling a task. It takes up contact by itself or refuses to do so if it feels displeasure. It allows itself to be distracted if one adapts to the child's needs/desires.

It already plays nicely with other children and defends its sphere of activity. It likes to play with adults as well.

Routines of Daily Life

The child's bladder control improves. It begins to make its needs known (there are differences between boys and girls, whereby girls are potty-trained earlier). The child eats at the table with the adults and uses a spoon to eat cut-up food. It drinks from a cup and is very proud

18

of its abilities, which makes it difficult to feed the child at all any more. It eats bread by itself without too much smearing.

The child undresses but does not yet dress by itself, although it tries to. It helps its mother with small household chores. The child's urge to expand can be somewhat dangerous and requires the adult's increased attention; however, the adult should be careful not to interfere too much. At this point, decisive feedback mechanisms arise which are vital for the child's further development.

Development

The child is considerably stable and capable of moving with good balance. Standing and hopping on one leg are not yet possible as stability is not pronounced enough for this yet. It tries to get to know its surroundings, takes up contact with persons, and touches everything, making it necessary to watch the child constantly. There are good intermediate stages of movements. It can squat and walks up and down stairs (holding onto something).

Its perceptual integration improves consistently. Its speech development corresponds to the development of motoricity which has taken place, i.e. sensorimotor adaptation, so that the child may now experience further dimensions of development.

Handling

(Tips for routine infant care which the doctor can show the mother.)

Before being able to walk about freely, all children are intensively subjected to the mother's handling. In children that display deviations in their motor development, that handling can have considerable influence on the child's further development. Since not only the child adapts to the mother's handling but also the mother reacts to faulty child behavior, it is possible and common for a mutual intensification and deepening of false child movement patterns to arise.

For example, if the child displays poor head control, the mother intuitively tends to support the child's head with her hand. Since the child then consistently receives help, it has difficulty to learn spontaneously how to improve its head control. Thus, the child's development is delayed due to the mother's handling.

Proper execution of the daily handling routines shown in the following pictures seems important, especially when dealing with a hypertonic child with persistent tonic posture patterns. The phenomena of hypertonus can become more pronounced if faulty handling is applied.

Daily routines such as bathing, feeding, carrying, and putting to bed are all manipulations that have considerable therapeutic value for a handicapped child and should not be underestimated. Using the following pictures, the normal handling of infants is briefly demonstrated.

These are only a few examples to use in order to influence the child's motoricity and psyche.

Carrying the child on the mother's body means transmitting her body image onto the child. This close contact gives the child security and a feeling of being cared for. This holds especially true for children that display difficulties maintaining an upright position.

"Handling" is also part of the treatment for more seriously afflicted children. At this point the reader's attention is directed to the book by Nancie R. Finnie entitled, *Handling the Young Cerebral Palsied Child at Home,* second edition, 1974, William Heinemann Medical Books Ltd., London.

There are two further handling methods which are likely to be important for the early phases of development and which are not used frequently enough as "handling" and/or therapeutic techniques, although they are probably of substantial value for cognitive and speech development.

One of these is caressing, which involves intensive skin contact, and the other is rocking and swinging (Figs. **159–197**).

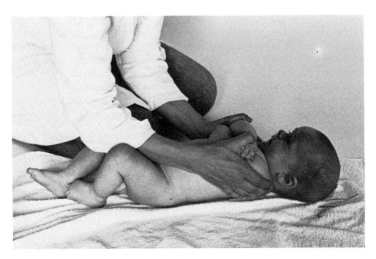

Fig. **159** When picking the child up, one should grasp the child at the shoulders using both hands and not pull it up by the arms

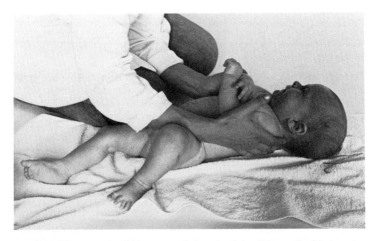

Fig. **160** The arms should be crossed since by doing this one is able to get a firm hold on the child. At the same time, one helps to prevent too much extension of the shoulders (shoulder retraction)

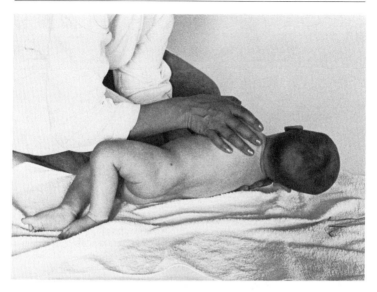

Fig. **161**   Pick up the child by rolling it over on one side. This rotation can help to improve head control

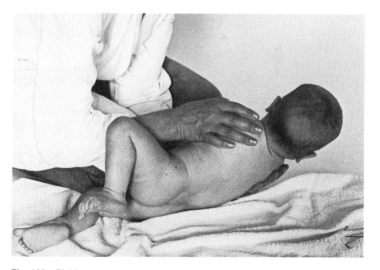

Fig. **162**   Picking up a child property

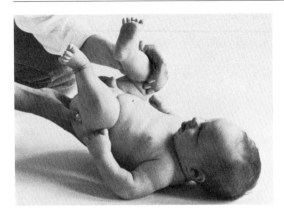

Fig. **163**   If one wishes to make the child's arms come forward without touching them so that the child touches its outer extremities, one must lift up its buttocks, holding the legs abducted and outwardly rotated. Always maintain eye contact and talk with the child

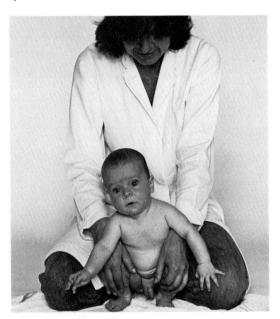

Fig. **164**   With the help of this position, head control can be improved; the child is in a symmetrical position. The shoulders are pushed forward. Retraction is not possible

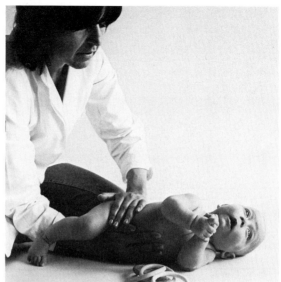

Fig. **165**

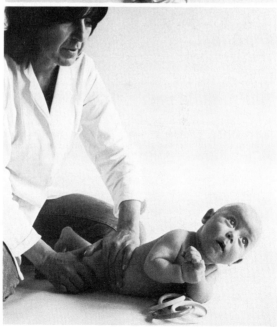

Fig. **166**

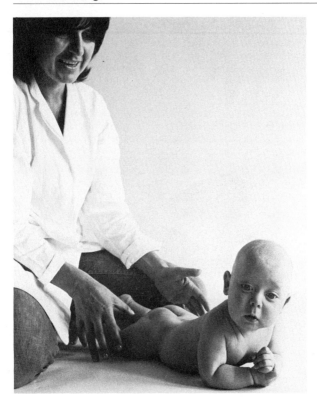

Fig. **167**

Figs. **165–167** In order to turn a child over from the supine to the prone position, it is not necessary to pick it up. One can turn the child by rolling it over at the hips

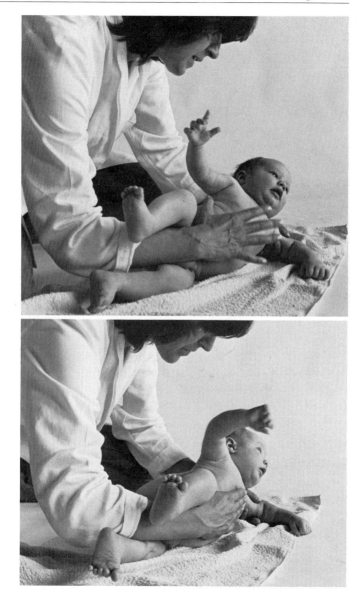

Figs. **168, 169**   Another possibility is to turn the child by putting pressure on its thorax, which makes rotation possible

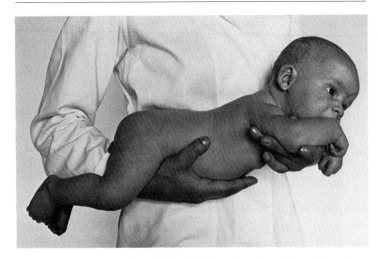

Fig. **170**   One can carry the child in a horizontal position. The mother places her arm between the child's legs so that her hand supports the thorax and abdomen. The other arm holds the child's arms forward as well as its shoulders

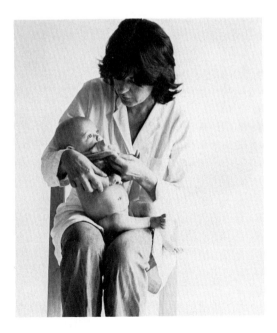

Fig. **171**

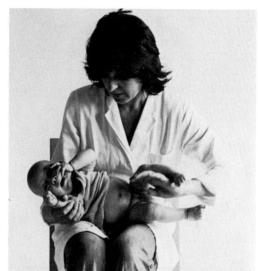

Figs. **172, 173**

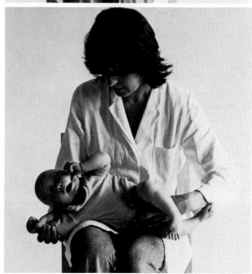

Figs. **171–173** Here, the possibility is demonstrated for dressing a child while it is on its mother's lap so that it does not lie on its back (as is usually the case), thus attaining extensive stretching and asymmetry. The child in these pictures is probably crying because it is lying "too high" (visual obstacle). This should always be taken into consideration

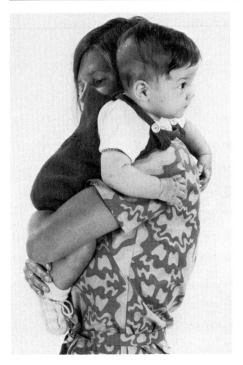

Fig. **174** If the child displays too much shoulder retraction, it can be carried as shown here, alternately resting on one of the mother's shoulders with its arms facing forward

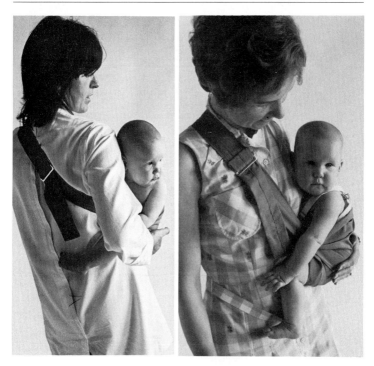

Figs. **175, 176** Carrying the child in a carrying shawl or wrap: the child's legs are abducted, while the head is not supported and is able to stabilize itself this way. The mother still has one hand free

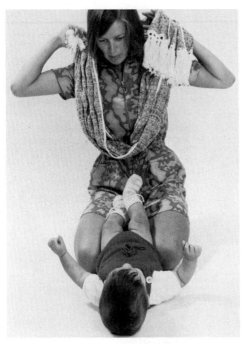

Figs. **177, 178**

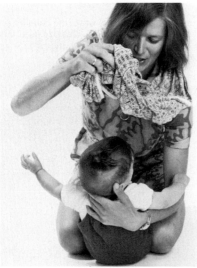

Figs. **177–181** Putting a carrying shawl around the child

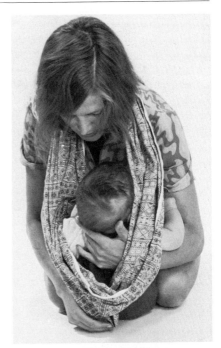

Fig. **179**

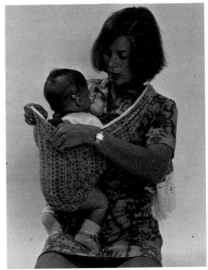

Fig. **180**

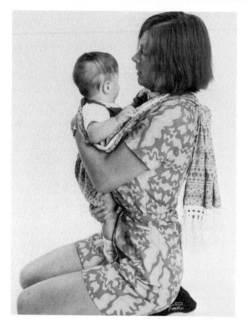

Fig. **181**

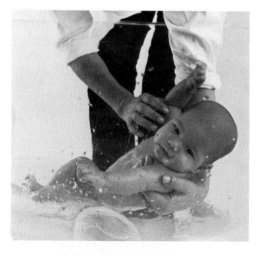

Fig. **182**

Figs. **182–184**   Bathing an infant in both the supine and the prone positions

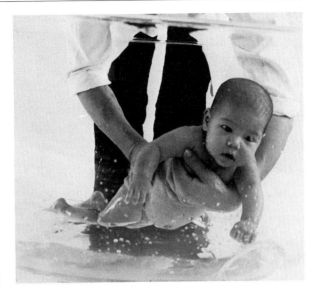

Fig. **183**

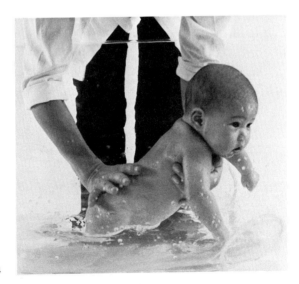

Fig. **184**

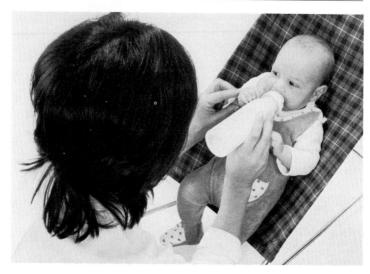

Fig. **185** Bottle-feeding a child in an infant seat. Symmetrical posture and eye contact

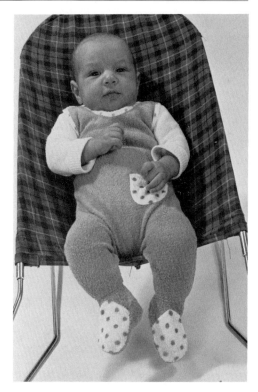

Fig. **186**   Symmetrical posture a child displays after having been set into an infant seat several times a day for 10–20 min. Good eye contact

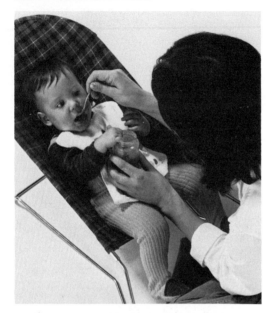

Fig. **187** Feeding an infant in an infant seat. Open hands, eye contact

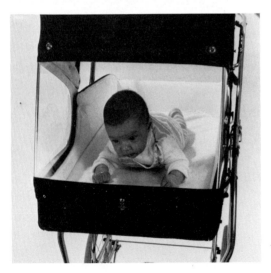

Fig. **188** Lying in a baby buggy. Head control in the prone position

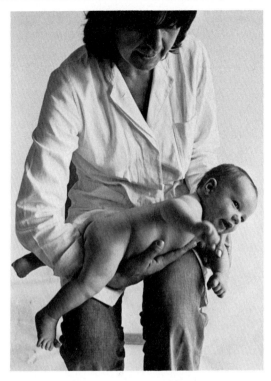

Fig. **189**   One possibility of carrying a child (extension)

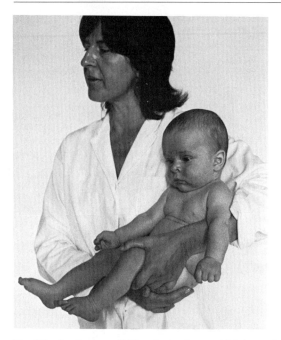

Fig. **190**   Another possibility of carrying a child (arms forward, good head control)

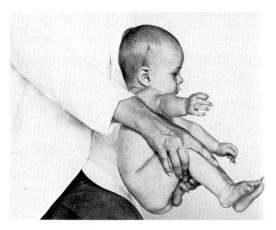

Fig. **191**   Still another possibility of carrying a child (symmetry, arms forward, hip abduction, head control)

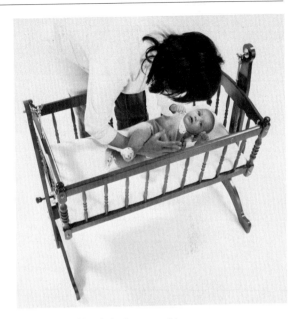

Fig. **192**   Position in bed on one side

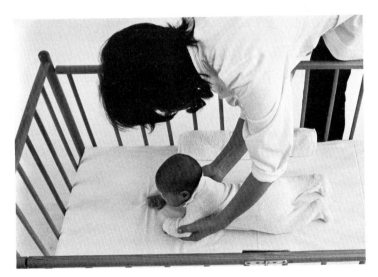

Fig. **193**   Prone position in bed

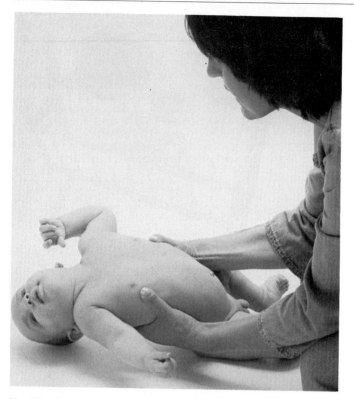

Fig. **194**   One example of how a child should not be picked up

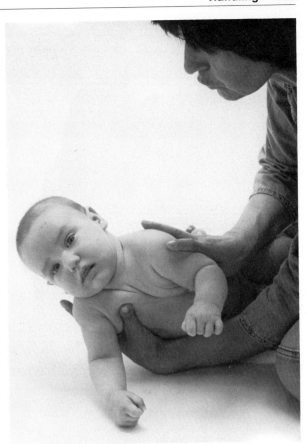

Fig. **195** Suggestion as to how a child could be picked up

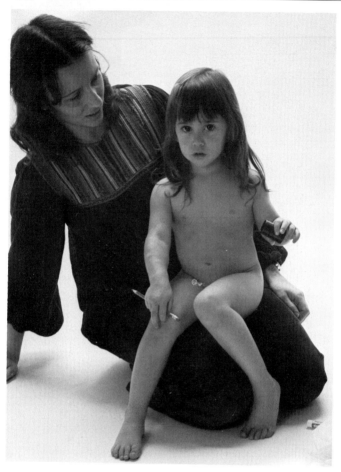

Fig. **196** Knock knee position

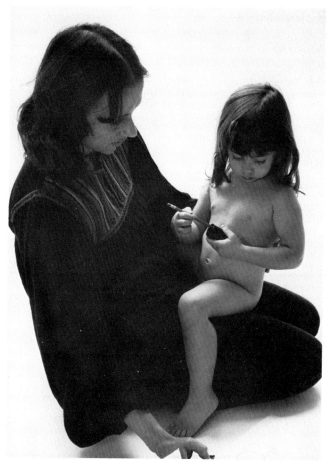

Fig. **197** Suggestion for positioning a child in order to correct the knock knees

References

Aebi, U.: Das normalbegabte zerebral bewegungsgestörte Kind. Huber, Bern, 1974a

Aebi, U.: Früherfassung der zerebralen Bewegungsstörungen. Pädiat. Fortbild. Prax. 40 (1974b) Sp. 64–73

Aebi, U., U. Wälti: Funktion und Grenzen der Frühpädagogik beim Kind mit zerebraler Bewegungsstörung. Pädiat. Fortbild. Prax. 40 (1974)

Agassiz, C. D. S., M. B. Oidonell, E. Collis: Early diagnosis of cerebral palsy. Lancet 1949/IV, 1030

Alcock, N. S.: The nature of paresis in cerebral palsy. In: Child Neurology and Cerebral Palsy. Little Club Clinics, Nr. 2. Heinemann, London 1960

Amiel-Tison, C.: Neurological evaluation of the maturity of newborn infants. Arch. Dis. Childh. 43 (1968) 89–93

Amiel-Tison, C., A. Grenier: Evaluation neurologique du nouveau-né et du nourrisson. (Neurological evaluation of the newborn and the nursing child.) Masson, Paris 1980

Anderson, U., M. R. Jenss, W. E. Mosher, C. L. Randall, E. Marra: High risk groups-definition and identification. New Engl. J. Med. 273 (1965) 308

André-Thomas, F. Hanon: Les premiers automatismes. Rev. neurol. 79 (1947) 641–648

André-Thomas, S. Saint-Anne Dargassies: Études Neurologiques sur le Nouveau-né et le Jeune Nourrisson. Masson & Perrin, Paris 1952

André-Thomas, Y. Chesni, S. Saint-Anne Dargassies: The Neurological Examination of the Infant. Little Club Clinics in Developmental Medicine, Nr. 1. Heinemann, London 1960

Ashby, W. R.: An Introduction to Cybernetics. Chapman and Hall, London, 1956

Ayres, Jean A.: Improving academic scores through sensory integration. J. Learn. Disab. 5 (1972) 24–28

Ayres, Jean A.: Learning disabilities and vestibular system. J. Learn. Disab. 11 (1978) 18–29

Ayres, Jean A.: Sensory Integration and Learning Disorders. Western Psychological Services, Los Angeles 1973

Ayres, Jean A.: Sensory Integration and the Child, Western Psychological Services, Los Angeles 1979/1980

Balduzzi, O.: Die Stützreaktionen beim Menschen in physiologischen und pathologischen Zuständen. Z. Neurol. 141 (1932) 1–29

Baver, J.: Das Kriechphänomen des Neugeborenen. Klin. Wschr. 5 (1926) 1468

Bax, M.: Terminology and classification of cerebral palsy. Develop. Med. Child Neurol. 6 (1964) 295

Bax, M. C. O., R. C. Mac Keith: Treatment of cerebral palsy. Develop. Med. Child Neurol. 15 (1973) 1

Bayley, N.: Bayley Scales of Infant Development. Psychological Corporation, New York 1969

Beintema, D. J.: A Neurological Study of New Born Infants. Clinics in Developmental Medicine, Nr. 28. Heinemann, London 1968

Bernuth, H. von: Die Frühdiagnose der infantilen Cerebralparese. Forschung und Praxis. Med. Welt 23 (N. F.) (1972) 442

Bobath, B.: A study of abnormal postural reflex activity in patients with lesions of the central nervous system. Physiotherapy (1954)

Bobath, B.: Observations on adult hemiplegia and suggestions for treatment. Physiotherapy (1960)

Bobath, B.: The Motor Disorders of Hemiplegia and their Physiotherapy. Little Club Clinics in Developmental Medicine, Nr. 4. Heinemann, London 1961 (S. 63)

Bobath, B.: Die Grundlagen der Behandlung des cerebral gelähmten Kindes. Pädiat. Fortbild. Prax. (1962) 61

Bobath, B.: A neuro-developmental treatment of cerebral palsy. Physiotherapy 47 (1963a)

Bobath, B.: Treatment principles and planning in cerebral palsy. Physiotherapy 47 (1963b)

Bobath, B.: The very early treatment of cerebral palsy. Develop. Med. Child Neurol. 9 (1967) 373–390

Bobath, B.: Abnorme Haltungsreflexe bei Gehirnschäden. Thieme, Stuttgart 1968, 3. Aufl. 1976

Bobath, B.: The treatment of neuromuscular disorders by improving patterns of co-ordination. Physiotherapy (1969)

Bobath, B.: Die neurologische Entwicklungsbehandlung des zerebral gelähmten Kindes. Materia med. Nordmark 22 (1970) 372

Bobath, B.: Motor development, its effect on general development, an application to the treatment of cerebral palsy. Physiotherapy (1971) 1

Bobath, B., K. Bobath: An analysis of the development of standing and walking patterns in patients with cerebral palsy. Physiotherapy 36 (1952)

Bobath, B., K. Bobath: Control of motor function in the treatment of cerebral palsy. Physiotherapy 41 (1957)

Bobath, B., K. Bobath: Grundgedanken zur Behandlung der zerebralen Kinderlähmung. Beitr. Orthop. Traum. 11 (1964) 225–251

Bobath, B., K. Bobath: Motor Development in the Different Types of Cerebral Palsy. Heinemann, London 1975

Bobath, B., E. Cotton: A patient with residual hemiplegia (and his respons to treatment). J. Amer. phys. Ther. Ass. 45 (1965) 849–864

Bobath, B., N. Finnie: Re-Education of movement patterns for everyday life in the treatment of cerebral palsy. Occup. Ther. J. (1958)

Bobath, K.: The neuropathology of cerebral palsy and its importance in treatment and diagnosis. Cerebr. Palsy Bull. 1 (1959) 13–33

Bobath, K.: The effect of treatment by reflex-inhibition and facilitation of movement in cerebral palsy. Folia psychiat. neer. 62 (1959) Nr. 5

Bobath, K.: The Nature of the Paresis In Cerebral Palsy. Second National Spastics Society Study Group, Oxford 1960

Bobath, K.: Two views on the tonic neck reflex. Develop. Med. Child Neurol. 4 (1962a) 220

Bobath, K.: The neurophysiology of cerebral palsy. Pädiat. Fortbild. Prax. (1962b) 48

Bobath, K.: The prevention of mental retardation in patients with cerebral palsy. Acta paedo Psychiat. 30 (1963) 141

Bobath, K.: Die Neuropathologie der zerebralen Kinderlähmung. In: Neurologie der Wirbelsäule und des Rückenmarks, hrsg. von D. Müller. Fischer, Jena 1964

Bobath, K.: Motor deficit in patients with cerebral palsy. Clinics in Developmental Medicine, No. 23, Spastics Society. Heinemann, London 1966

Bobath, K.: Die Neuropathologie der infantilen Zerebralparese. In: Diagnostik und Therapie zerebraler Bewegungsstörungen im Kindesalter. Bartmann, Frechen 1969 (S. 83–112)

Bobath, K.: Eine moderne Behandlung der zerebralen Bewegungsstörung und ihre Bedeutung für die körperliche und geistige Entwicklung des Kindes. Materia med. Nordmark 22 (1970) 364

Bobath, K.: Frühbehandlung und ihre methodischen Grundlagen. In: Spastisch gelähmte Kinder, hrsg. von H. H. Matthias, H. T. Brüster, H. v. Zimmermann. Thieme, Stuttgart 1971 (S. 173–178)

Bobath, K.: Die normale motorische Entwicklung des Kindes während des ersten Lebensjahres und ihre Abweichungen bei infantiler Zerebralparese. In: Spastisch gelähmte Kinder, hrsg. von H. H. Matthias, H. T. Brüster, H. v. Zimmermann. Thieme, Stuttgart 1971

Bobath, K.: Entwicklung des Konzeptes des „Neurodevelopmental Treatment". Pädiat. Fortbild. Prax. 40 (1974a) 97–100

Bobath, K.: Klassische Bilder im Lichte moderner Diagnostik. Pädiat. Fortbild. Prax. 40 (1974b) 1–12

Bobath, K.: Erfahrungen mit zerebralparetischen, schwer geistig behinderten Kindern. Pädiat. Fortbild. Prax. 40 (1974c) 194–197

Bobath, K., B. Bobath: The diagnosis of cerebral palsy in infancy. Arch. Dis. Childh. 31 (1956) 408

Bobath, K., B. Bobath: An assessment of the motor handicap of children with cerebral palsy and of their response to treatment. Occup. Ther. J. (1958)

Bobath, K., B. Bobath: Grundgedanken zur Behandlung der zerebralen Kinderlähmung. Beitr. Orthop. Traum. 8 (1961). H. 3

Bobath, K., B. Bobath: The facilitation of normal postural reactions and movements in the treatment of cerebral palsy. Physiotherapy 48 (1964)

Brandt, S.: Very early treatment of cerebral palsy (Letters to the Editor). Develop. Med. Child Neurol. 8 (1966) 353–354

Brazelton, T. B.: Babys erstes Lebensjahr. Maier, Ravensburg 1969

Brazelton, T. B.: Assessment of infant at risk. Clin. Obstet. a. Gynec. 16 (1973) 361–375

Brazelton, T. B.: Neonatal Behavioural Assessment Scale. Clinics in Developmental Medicine, Nr. 50. Heinemann, London 1973

Bruner, J. S.: The growth and structure of skill. In: Mechanisms of Motor Skill Development, hrsg. von K. Conolly. Academic Press, London 1970 (S. 63–92)

Bruner, J. S.: Organization of early skilled action. Child Develop 44 (1973a) 1–11

Bruner, J. S.: Relevanz der Erziehung. Otto-Maier-Verlag, Ravensburg 1973b

Bryant, Gillian M., Kathleen J. Davies, F. Marie Richards, Susan Voorhees: A preliminary study of the use of the Denver Developmental Screening Test in a Health Department. Develop. Med. Child Neurol. 15 (1973) 33

Bryant, Gillian M., Kathleen J. Davies: The effect of sex, social class and parity on achievement of Denver Developmental Screening Test items in the first year of life. Develop. Med. Child Neurol. 16 (1974) 485

Bryant, Gillian M., Kathleen J. Davies, Robert Newcombe: The Dever Developmental Screening Test. Achievement of Test items in the first year of life by Denver and Cardiff infants. Develop. Med. Child Neurol. 16 (1974) 475

Byers, R. K.: Tonic neck reflexes in children considered from a prognostic standpoint. Amer. J. Dis. Child 55 (1938) Nr. 4

Casaer, P., E. Eggermont: Neonatal clinical neurological assessment. In: The At-Risk Infant, hrsg. von S. Harel, N. Anastasiow. Brookes, Baltimore 1985; dt. Übersetzung in: Kindesentwicklung und Lernverhalten, hrsg. von I. Flehmig, L. Stern. Fischer, Stuttgart 1986 (S. 121–154)

Chapman, S.: Sensori-motor stimulation for the young handicapped child. Develop. Med. Child Neurol. 16 (1974) 546

Chee, F. K. W., J. R. Kreutzberg, D. L. Clark: Semicircular canal stimulation in cerebral palsied children. Phys. Ther. 58 (1978) 1017–1075

Christian, P.: Studien zur Willkürmotorik. I. über die Objektbildung in der Motorik. Dtsch. Z. Nervenheilk. 167 (1952) 237

Christian, P.: Über „Leistungsanalyse", dargestellt an Beispielen aus der Willkürmotorik. Nervenarzt 24 (1953) 10–16

Christian, P.: Möglichkeiten und Grenzen einer naturwissenschaftlichen Betrachtung der menschlichen Bewegung. Jb. Psychol. u. Psychother. 4 (1956) 346–356

Clark, D. L., J. R. Kreutzberg, F. K. W. Chee: Vestibular stimulation influence on motor development in infants. Science 196 (1977) 1228–1229

Collis, Eirene: Some differential characteristics of cerebral motor defects in infancy. Arch. Dis. Childh. 29 (1964) 113–122

Denhoff, E., R. H. Holden: Etiology of cerebral palsy. An experimental approach. Amer. J. Obstet. Gynec. 70 (1955) 274–281

Denhoff, E., R. H. Holden, M. L. Silver: Prognostic studies in children with cerebral palsy. J. Amer. med. Ass. 161 (1956) 781–784

Dobler, H.-J.: Biologische Reifung der neurologischen und stato-motorischen Entwicklung. Fortschr. Med. 88 (1970) Nr. 1

Dubowitz, L. M. S.: Neurological assessment of the full-term and preterm newborn infant. In: The At-Risk Infant, Edt. S. Harel, N. Anastasiow. Brookes, Baltimoore 1985, p. 185–196

Dubowitz, L. M. S., V. Dubowitz: The Neurological Assessment of the Preterm and Full-term Newborn Infant. Clinics in Developmental Medicine, Nr. 79. Heinemann, London 1981

Dudenhausen, J. W., E. Saling: Risikoschwangerschaft und Risikogeburt. Materia med. Nordmark 67 (1974)

Egan, D. F., R. S. Illingworth, R. C. Mackeith: Developmental screening 0–5 years. Clinics in Developmental Medicine, Nr. 30. Heinemann, London 1971

Eggert, D., E. J. Kiphard: Die Bedeutung der Motorik für die Entwicklung normaler und behinderter Kinder. Hoffmann, Schorndorf b. Stuttgart 1973

Ellis, E.: The Physical Management of Developmental Disorders. Heinemann, London 1967

Feldkamp, Margaret: Was wird aus den frühdiagnostizierten und frühbehandelten Kindern mit „cerebraler Bewegungsstörung"? Krankengymnastik 11 (1972a) 345–346

Feldkamp, Margaret: Frühdiagnostik der cerebralen Bewegungsstörungen bei Frühgeborenen. Pädiat. Fortbild. Prax. 32 (1972b) 62–74

Feldkamp, M., J. Danielcik: Krankengymnastische Behandlung der cerebralen Bewegungsstörung. Pflaum, München 1973

Finnie, Nancie R.: Hilfe für das cerebral gelähmte Kind. Maier, Ravensburg 1976

Flehmig, I.: Praktische Hinweise zur Früherkennung cerebraler Bewegungsstörungen im Hinblick auf eine neurophysiologische Behandlung. Mschr. Kinderheilk. 117 (1969) 641–644

Flehmig, I.: Statisch-motorische Entwicklung des Säuglings und Kleinkindes. In: Handbuch der Kinderheilkunde, Bd. I/1, hrsg. von H. Opitz, F. Schmid. Springer, Berlin 1971

Flehmig, I.: Der „Denver-Suchtest" als Screeningmethode. Kinderarzt 2 (1972) 61–63

Flehmig, I.: Früherkennung zerebraler Bewegungsstörungen. Materia med. Nordmark 67 (1974) 3–20

Flehmig, I.: Die Denver Entwicklungsskalen (DES). In: Frühe Hilfen – wirksamste Hilfen, hrsg. von der Bundesvereinigung Lebenshilfe für geistig Behinderte e. V., Bundeszentrale, Marburg 1975

Flehmig, I.: Nachuntersuchungen im Hinblick auf Diagnose und Therapie der zerebralen Bewegungsstörungen. Krankengymnastik 29 (1977) 10–14

Flehmig, I., H. Wiesener: Auftreten und Wertigkeit von Frühsymptomen cerebraler Bewegungsstörungen bei Frühgeborenen und Reifgeborenen der Gefahrengruppe. Mschr. Kinderheilk. 116 (1968) 323–325

Frank, Lawrence K.: Tactile communication. Genet. Psychol. Monogr. 56 (1957) 209–225

Frankenburg, W. K., J. B. Dodds: Denver developmental screening test. J. Pediat. 71 (1967) 181–191

Frankenburg, W. K., B. W. Camp, P. A. van Natta: Validity of the Denver developmental screening test. Child Develop. 42 (1971a) 475–485

Frankenburg, W. K., A. D. Goldstein, B. Camp: The revised Denver developmental screening test: its accuracy as a screening instrument. J. Pediat. 79 (1971b) 988–995

Freud, S.: Zur Kenntnis der cerebralen Diplegien des Kindesalters. Leipzig 1893

Freud, S.: Die infantile Cerebrallähmung. In: Spezielle Pathologie und Therapie, Bd. IX/3, hrsg. von H. Nothnagel, Wien 1901

Funke, W.: Die klinisch „diskrete" Frühkindliche Encephalopathie – Gedanken zur diagnostischen therapeutischen und sozialprognostischen Problematik. Mschr. Kinderheilk. 114 (1966) H. 8

Galant, S.: Der Rückgratreflex. Dissertation, Basel 1917

Gesell, A.: The tonic reflex in human infant. J. Pediat. 13 (1938) 455

Gesell, A.: The First Five Years of Life. Harper & Row, New York 1940

Gesell A., C. Amatruda: Developmental Diagnosis Normal and Abnormal Child Development. Hoeber, New York 1941 u. 1949

Gibson, James J.: Die Sinne und der Prozeß der Wahrnehmung. Huber, Bern (1973)

Göb, A.: Die fortlaufende Überprüfung der frühkindlichen Hirnschäden an der motorischen Entwicklung und dem Reflexverhalten. Z. Orthop. 103 (1967) 221–240

Golay, L.: Les handicaps associés des infirmités motrices cérébrales. Pädiat. Fortbild. Prax. 2 (1962) 26

Goldman, P. S.: The role of experience in recovery of function following orbital prefrontal lesions in infant monkeys. Neuropsychologica 14 (1976) 401–411

Girant, W., A. N. Boelsche, D. Zin: Developmental patterns of two motor functions. Develop. Med. Child Neurol. 15 (1973) 171

Gressmann, C.: Dissoziierte Entwicklungsparameter bei Frühgeborenen mit Spastischer Cerebralparese. Z. Orthop. 103 (1967) 543 f.

Gressmann, Christine: Dokumentation in der Behandlung des zerebralparetischen Kindes. In: Schriftenreihe der medizinisch-orthopädischen Technik, Bd. II. Gentner, Stuttgart 1976

Griffiths, R.: The Abilities of Babies. University of London Press, London 1954

Grossmann, K. E.: Entwicklung der Lernfähigkeit in der sozialen Umwelt. Kindler-Taschenbücher 2177. Kindler, München 1977

Hagberg, B.: Klinische Syndrome bei Cerebralparese. Mschr. Kinderheilk. 121 (1973) 259–264

Hagberg, B., A. Lundberg: Dissociated motor development simulating cerebral palsy. Neuropädiatrie 1 (1969) 187

Hagberg, B., G. Sauner, M. Steen: The Dysequilibrium Syndrom. In Cerebral Palsy. Almquist & Wiksell, Uppsala 1972

Hellbrügge, T., J. Pechstein: Entwicklungsphysiologische Tabellen für das Säuglingsalter. Fortschr. Med. Heft 86 (1968); rev. Ausgabe 11 und 14, 1969

Hellbrügge, Th., I. H. v. Wimpffen: Die ersten 365 Tage im Leben eines Kindes. Die Entwicklung des Säuglings. TR-Verlagsunion, München 1975

Herbinet, E., M.-C. Busnel: L'Aube des Sens, Les Cahiers du Nouveau-Né No. 5 Editions Stock, Paris 1981

Herschkowitz, N.: Normale und abnorme Entwicklung der Gehirnstrukturen. Pädiat. Fortbild. Prax. 40 (1974)

Hochleitner, Margit: Zerebrale Bewegungsstörungen. Mitt. öst. Sanit.-Verwalt. 69 (1968) 2

Hochleitner, M.: Pathologische Haltungs- und Bewegungsmuster beim zerebralparetischen Säugling. Fortschr. Med. 87 (1969) 1091–1097

Hochleitner, M., H. Berger: Cerebrale Bewegungsstörung – Untersuchungsmethoden. F. d. M.-Tabellen für die Praxis, 17. Verlag Fortschritte der Medizin, Gauting 1966

Holden, R. H., G. Solomons: Relations between pediatrics, psychological, and neurological examinations during the first year of life. Child. Develop. 33 (1962) 719

Holt, K. S.: Early motor development. J. Pediat. 57 (1960) 571–575

Holt, K. S.: Assessment of Cerebral Palsy. Lloyd-Luke, London 1965

Hoskins, T. A., J. E. Squires: Developmental assessment: A test for gross motor and reflex development. Phys. Ther. 53 (1973) 117–126

Huth, E.: Die Frühdiagnose der infantilen Cerebral-Parese. Arch. Kinderheilk. 170 (1964) 110–125

Huth, E.: Die Prophylaxe frühkindlicher Hirnschäden. Die Folgezustände frühkindlicher Hirnschäden aus pädiatrischer Sicht. In: Die Prophylaxe frühkindlicher Hirnschäden, hrsg. von R. Elert, K. A. Hüter. Thieme, Stuttgart 1966 (S. 15–26)

Illingworth, R. S.: Early Diagnosis and Differential Diagnosis. III: The Diagnosis of cerebral palsy. In: Recent Advances in Cerebral Palsy. Churchill, London 1958a (S. 46–63)

Illingworth, R. S.: Early diagnosis of cerebral palsy. Cerebr. Palsy Bull. 2 (1958b) 6

Illingworth, R. S.: An introduction to developmental assessment in the first year. Little Club Clinics in Developmental Medicine, Nr. 3. Heinemann, London 1962

Illingworth, R. S.: The Development of the Infant and Young Child – Normal and Abnormal. Livingstone, Edinburgh 1966

Illingworth, R. S.: Die Diagnose der Zerebralparese im ersten Lebensjahr. In: Spastisch gelähmte Kinder, hrsg. von H. H. Matthiass, H. T. Brüster, H. v. Zimmermann. Thieme, Stuttgart 1971

Ingram, T. T. S.: The early manifestation and course of diplegia in childhood. Arch. Dis. Childh. 30 (1955) 244

Ingram, T. T. S.: Muscle tone and posture in infancy. Cerebral Palsy Bull. 5 (1959) 6–15

Ingram, T. T. S.: Clinical significance of the infantile feeding reflexes. Develop. Med. Child Neurol. 4 (1962) 159–169

Ingram, T. T. S.: The neurology of cerebral palsy. Arch. Dis. Childh. 41 (1966) 337–355

Ingram, T. T. S.: The new approach to early diagnosis of handicaps in childhood. Develop. Med. Child Neurol. 11 (1969) 279–290

Ingram, T. T. S.: Soft signs. Develop. Med. Child Neurol. 15 (1973) 527

Isaacson, R. L.: The myth of recovery from early brain damage. In Ellis, N. R.: Aberrant Development of Infancy, Potomac, Md.: Lawrence Erlbaum Associates, 1975

Jackson, J. H.: In: Selected Writings of John Highling Jackson, Bd. I u. II, hrsg. von J. Taylor. Basic Books, New York 1958

Jantzen, Wolfgang: Menschliche Entwicklung, Allgemeine Pädagogik. Jarick, Solms-Oberbiel 1980

Jetter, K.: Kindliches Handeln und kognitive Entwicklung. Huber, Bern 1975

Johnson, D. J., H. R. Myklebust: Lernschwächen. Hippokrates, Stuttgart 1971

Jones, B.: The importance of memory traces of motor efferent discharges for learning skilled movements. Develop. Med. Child Neurol. 16 (1974) 620

Joppich, G., F. J. Schulte: Neurologie des Neugeborenen. Springer, Berlin 1968

Kennard, M. A.: Value of equivocal signs in neurologic diagnosis. Neurology (Minneap.) 10 (1960) 753

Knobloch, H., B. Pasamanick, E. S. Sherard: A developmental screening inventory for infants. Pediatrics 38 (1966) 1095

Köng, E.: Frühdiagnose zerebraler Lähmungen. Pädiat. Fortbild. Prax. 1 (1962a) 37

Köng, E.: Behandlungsresultate bei Früh- und Spätfällen. Pädiat. Fortbild. Prax. 24 (1962b) 68

Köng, E.: Minimal cerebral palsy: The importance of its recognition. Little Club Clinics in Developmental Medicine, Nr. 10. Heinemann, London 1963a, (S. 29)

Köng, E.: Cerebrale Lähmungen: Orthopädisch-neurologische Grenzprobleme. Pädiat. Fortbild. Prax. 5/6 (1963b) 103–110

Köng, E.: Frühdiagnose und Frühbehandlung cerebraler Bewegungsstörungen („Lähmungen") mit Demonstration von Behandlungsresultaten. Praxis 54 (1965) 1280–1284

Köng, E.: Very early treatment of cerebral palsy. Develop. Med. Child Neurol. 8 (1966a) 206–209

Köng, E.: Frühbehandlung cerebraler Bewegungsstörungen unter Mitarbeit der Eltern. Pädiat. Pädol. 2, H. 2/3 (1966b) Sonderdruck (nicht im Handel)

Köng, E.: Erfahrungen mit der Frühbehandlung zerebraler Bewegungsstörungen. In: Verhandlungen der Deutschen Orthopädischen Gesellschaft, 54. Kongreß, hrsg. von M. Lange. Enke, Stuttgart 1967

Köng, E.: Die Frühbehandlung cerebraler Bewegungsstörungen. Mschr. Kinderheilk. 116 (1968) 281–284

Köng, E.: Früherfassung zerebraler Bewegungsstörungen. Pädiat. Fortbild. Prax. 33 (1972) 1ff.

Köng, E.: Erfahrungen mit der Frühtherapie. Pädiat. Fortbild. Prax. 40 (1974a) 132–137

Köng, E.: Aspekte des Sportes bei zerebralen Bewegungsstörungen. Pädiat. Fortbild. Prax. 40 (1974b) 164–168

Köng, E.: Cerebrale Bewegungsstörung heute: Probleme der Diagnostik-Möglichkeiten und Grenzen der Behandlung (nicht veröffentlicht)

Köng, E., A. Lynn: Erfahrungen mit langjähriger Therapie spätbehandelter Kinder. Pädiat. Fortbild. Prax. 40 (1974) 104–126

Köng, E., J. Nichil, A. Grenier: La Kinésithérapie des I. M. C.-possibilités et limites. Bull. Inf. mot. cer., Suppl., 56 (1970)

Köng, E., R. Tobler, Z. Birò: Erfassung cerebraler Bewegungsstörungen bei Frühgeborenen. Praxis 57 (1968) 1530–1533

Korner, A. F., E. B. Thoman: The relative efficacy of contact and vestibular-proprioceptive stimulation in soothing neonates. Child. Develop. 43 (1972) 443–453

Kressin, W., M. Rautenbach: Zerebrale Bewegungsstörungen im Kindesalter: Frühdiagnose, Grundzüge der Behandlung, Dispensaire Betreuung. VEB Volk und Gesundheit, Berlin 1976

Lajosi, F.: Erfahrungen mit schematisierten Untersuchungsprotokollen. In: Pädiatr. Fortbildungskurse 40. S. Karger, Basel 1974, Pädiat. Fortbild. Prax. 40 (1974) 78–87

Landau, A.: Über motorische Besonderheiten des zweiten Lebensjahres. Mschr. Kinderheilk. 29 (1925) 333

Landau, A.: Über einen tonischen Lagereflex beim Säugling. Klin. Wschr. 2 (1932) 1253–1255

Leboyer, Frédérick: Sanfte Hände. Kösel, München 1979

Lesigang, Ch.: Risikokinder. In: Jahrbuch für Jugendpsychiatrie und ihre Grenzgebiete, Bd. VIII 1971 (S. 105–121)

Little, W.: On the influence of abnormal parturition difficult labours, premature birth and asphyxia neonatorum, on the mental and physical conditions of the child. Cerebral Palsy Bull. (1958) 1; Trans. Obstet. Soc. Lond. 111 (1862) 293

Lübbe, C.: Erläuterungen über die Behandlung mit dem Lagerungsleibchen. Kinderarzt (1976) H. 5 568

Mac Keith, R.: The primary walking response and its facilitation by passive extension of the head. Acta paediat. Lat. (Reggio Emilia), (1964) 710

Mac Keith, R. C., J. C. K. Mac Kencie, P. E. Pocani: The Little Club Memorandum on Terminology and Classification of „Cerebral Palsy". Cerebr. Palsy Bull. 1 (1959) 27

Magnus, R.: Körperstellung. Springer, Berlin 1924

Magnus, R.: Physiology of posture. Lancet 1926/II, 5376

Magnus, R., de Kleijn: Die Abhängigkeit des Tonus der Extremitätenmuskulatur von der Kopfstellung. Pflügers Arch. ges. Physiol. 145 (1912) 455, 548

Matthiass, H.-H.: Untersuchungstechnik und Diagnose der Infantilen Zerebralparese im Säuglings- und Kindesalter. Thieme, Stuttgart 1966

McGraw, M. B.: The Neuromuscular Maturation of the Human Infant. Columbia University Press, New York 1943

Meitinger, Ch., V. Vlach, H. M. Weinmann: Neurologische Untersuchungen bei Frühgeborenen. Münch. med. Wschr. 111 (1969) 1158

Michaelis, R., R. Dopfer, W. Gerbig, P. Dopfer-Feller, M. Rohr: 1. Die Erfassung obstetrischer und postnataler Risikofaktoren durch die Liste optimaler Bedingungen. Mschr. Kinderheilk. 127 (1979) 149–155
2. Die Verteilung obstetrischer und postnataler Risikofaktoren bei 400 zufällig ausgewählten Neugeborenen. Mschr. Kinderheilk. 127 (1979) 196–200

Milani-Comparetti, A.: Spasticity versus patterned postural and motor behaviour of spastics. Proceedings of the IVth International Congress of Physical Medicine, Paris 1964

Milani-Comparetti, A.: The nature of motor disorders in cerebral palsy. Clin. Proc. (1967)

Milani-Comparetti, A.: Erfahrungen mit einem neuro-evolutiven Test. Pädiat. Fortbild. Prax. 40 (1974a) 74–77

Milani-Comparetti, A.: Klassifikation der physiotherapeutischen Behandlungsmethoden. Pädiat. Fortbild. Prax. 40 (1974b) 157–163

Milani-Comparetti, A.: La Terapia dell'affezioni neuromotorie infantili. In: Bonavita, V.: Terapia in neurologica (in Druck)

Milani-Comparetti, A., E. A. Gidoni: Pattern analysis of motor development and its disorders. Develop. Med. Child Neurol. 9 (1967a) 625–630

Milani-Comparetti, A., E. A. Gidoni: Routine developmental examination in normal and retarded children. Develop. Med. Child Neurol. 9 (1967b) 631

Milani-Comparetti, A., E. A. Gidoni: Significato della semeiotica reflessologica per la diagnosi neuroevolutiva. Neuropsychiat. Infant 121 (1971)

Milani-Comparetti, A., E. A. Gidoni: Dalla parte del neonato: Proposte per una competenza prognostica. Neuropsychiat. Infant 175 (1976) 5

Milani-Comparetti, A.: The neurophysiologic and clinical implications of studies on fetal motor behavior. Semin. Perinatol. 5 (1981) 183–189

Minear, W. L.: A classification of cerebral palsy. Pediatrics 18 (1956) 841–852

Montagu, Ashley: Körperkontakt. Klett, Stuttgart 1974

Moro, E.: Das erste Trimenon. Münch. med. Wschr. 65 (1918) 1147

Mosthaf, Ursula: Funktionelle Ergotherapie bei Kindern mit zerebralen Bewegungsstörungen. Pädiat. Fortbild. Prax. 40 (1974) 101–103

Müller, Helen A.: Vorbereitende Sprachtherapie. Pädiat. Fortbild. Prax. 40 (1974) 127–131

v. Muralt, G.: Perinatale Erfassung der Risikokinder. Pädiat. Fortbild. Prax. 40 (1974) 13–43

Narabayashi, H., M. Nagahata, T. Nagao, H. Shimazu: A new classification of cerebral palsy based upon neurophysiologic considerations. Confin. neurol. (Basel) 25 (1965) 378

Neligan, G., D. Prudham: Norms for four standard developmental milestones by sex, social class and place in family. Develop. Med. Child Neurol. 11 (1969) 413–422

Oettinger, L.: The asymmetrical tonic neck reflex. Develop. Med. Child Neurol. 17 (1975) 119

Oppé, T. E.: Risk registers for babies. Develop. Med. Child Neurol. 9 (1967) 13

Ottenbacher, Kenneth: Identifying vestibular processing dysfunktion in learning disabled children. Amer. J. occup. Ther. 32 (1978) 217–221

Paine, R. S.: The early diagnosis of cerebral palsy. R. I. med. J. 44 (1961) 522–527

Paine, R. S.: The evolution of infantile postural reflexes in the presence of chronic brain syndromes. Develop. Med. Child Neurol. 6 (1964) 345–361

Paine, R. S.: Early recognition of neuromotor disability in infant of low birthweight. Develop. Med. Child Neurol. 11 (1969) 455

Paine, R. S., T. E. Oppé: Die neurologische Untersuchung von Kindern. Thieme, Stuttgart 1970

Paine, R. S., T. B. Brazelton, D. E. Donovan, J. E. Rorbaugh, J. P. Hubbell jr., E. Manning Sears: Evolution of postural reflexes in normal infants and in the presence of chronic brain syndromes. Neurology (Minneap.) 14 (1964) 1037–1048

Papoušek, H.: Die Entwicklung früher Lernprozesse im Säuglingsalter. Kinderarzt 6 (1975) I 1077, II 1205, III 1331.

Parmelee, A. H., M. D. Michaelis: Neurological examination of the human newborn. In: Exceptional Infant, hrsg. von J. Hellmuth, Bd. II. Brunner/Mazel, New York 1971

Parmelee, A. H., F. J. Schulte: Developmental testing of pre-term and small-for-date infants. Pediatrics 45 (1970) 2128

Peiper, A.: Beiträge zur Neurologie des jungen Säuglings. Mschr. Kinderheilk. 45 (1931) 265

Peiper, A.: Das Stehen im Säuglingsalter. Jb. Kinderheilk. 134 (1932) 149

Peiper, A.: Instinkt und angeborenes Schema beim Säugling. Z. Tierpsychol. 8 (1951) 449–456

Peiper, A.: Eigenarten kindlicher Hirntätigkeit, 3. Aufl. Edition, Leipzig 1964

Peiper, A., H. Isbert: Über die Körperstellung des Säuglings. Jb. Kinderheilk. 115 (1927) 142–176

Perlstein, M. A.: Infantile cerebral palsy. J. Amer. med. Ass. 149 (1952) 30–34

Perlstein, M. A., H. E. Barnett: Nature and recognition of cerebral palsy in infancy. J. Amer. med. Ass. 148 (1952) 1389–1397

Pette, H.: Klinische und anatomische Studien zum Kapitel der tonischen Hals- und Labyrinthreflexe beim Menschen. Dtsch. Z. Nervenheilk. 86 (1925) 193

Phelps, W. M.: The management of the cerebral palsied. J. Amer. med. Ass. 117 (1941) 1621

Piaget, Jean: Das Erwachen der Intelligenz beim Kinde. Ges. Werke, Stud.-Ausgabe, Bd. I. Klett, Stuttgart 1975

Prechtl, H. F. R.: Über die Kopplung von Saugen und Greifen beim Säugling. Naturwissenschaften 40 (1953) 347

Prechtl, H. F. R.: Die Entwicklung und Eigenart frühkindlicher Bewegungsweisen. Klin. Wschr. 34 (1956) 281–284

Prechtl, H. F. R.: The directed head turning and allied movements of the human baby. Behaviour 13 (1958) 212–242

Prechtl, H. F. R.: Die neurologische Untersuchung des Neugeborenen. Voraussetzungen, Methode und Prognose. Wien. med. Wschr. 110 (1960a) 1035–1039

Prechtl. H. F. R.: The Long Term Value of the Neurological Examination of the Newborn Infant. The Second National Spastics Soc. Study Group, Oxford 1960b

Prechtl. H. F. R.: Prognostic value of neurological signs in the newborn infant. Proc. roy. Soc. Med. 58 (1965) 3–4

Prechtl, H. F. R.: Neurological findings in newborn infants after pre- and paranatal complications. In: Nutricia Symposium. Stenfert Kroese, Leiden 1968

Prechtl, H. F. R.: Hazards of oversimplification. Develop. Med. Child Neurol. 12 (1970) 522–524

Prechtl. H. F. R.: Strategy and validity of early detection of neurological dysfunction. In: Mental Retardation: Prenatal Diagnosis and Infant Assessment, hrsg. von C. P. Douglas, K. S. Holt. Butherworth, London 1972 (S. 41–47)

Prechtl, H. F. R.: The Neurological Examination of the Full-term Newborn Infant. Clinics in developmental Medicine, Nr. 63. Heinemann, London 1977

Prechtl, H. F. R., D. Beintema: The Neurological Examination of the Full Term Newborn Infant. Little Club Clinics in Developmental Medicine, No. 12. Heinemann, London 1964

Prechtl, H. F. R., D. J. Beintema: Die neurologische Untersuchung des Reifen Neugeborenen, 2. Aufl. Thieme, Stuttgart 1976

Prechtl, H. F. R.: The study of neural development as perspective of clinical problems. In Connolly, K. J., H. F. R. Prechtl.: Maturation and Development. Clinics in Developmental Medicine No. 77/78, London: William Heinemann Medical Books, Philadelphia: J. B. Lippincott Co., 1981

Rademaker, G. C. J.: Réactions Labyrinthiques et Equilibre. Masson, Paris 1935

Robinson, R. J.: Assessment of gestational age by neurological examination. Arch. Dis. Childh. 41 (1966) 437–447

Robson, P.: Persisting head turning in the early months: Some effects in the early years. Develop. Med. Child Neurol. 10 (1968) 82

Robson, P.: Variations of normal motor development. Paper read at the Study Group on Promoting Better Movement in Children with Motor Handicap. The Spastics Society, Nottingham 1973

Rogers, M. G. H.: Risk registers and early detection of handicaps. Develop. Med. Child Neurol. 10 (1968) 651–661

Saint-Anne Dargassies, S.: Méthode d'examen neurologique sur le nouveau-né. Étud. néo-natal. 3 (1954) 101

Saint-Anne Dargassies, S.: Maturation neurologique du prématuré. Étud. néo-natal. 4 (1955) 71

Saint-Anne Dargassies, S.: Les différents stades de la maturation neurologique du nourrisson normal et pathologique. Proceedings of the 2nd International Congress on Mental Retardation, Vienna 1961, Part I (S. 164)

Saint-Anne Dargassies, S.: Le nouveau-né à terme: aspect neurologique. Biol. neonat. 4 (1962) 174

Saint-Anne Dargassies, S.: Introduction à la sémiologie du développement neurologique du nourrisson normal. I. Conceptions générales. II. Méthode d'exploration neurologique. J. neurol. Sci. 1 (1964a) 160

Saint-Anne Dargassies, S.: Introduction à la sémiologie du développement neurologique du nourrisson normal. II. Méthode d'exploration neurologique. J. neurol. Sci. 1 (1964b) 578

Saint-Anne Dargassies, S.: Détection précoce des déficits chez le prématuré. Méd. Infant. 8 (1964c) 475

Saint-Anne Dargassies, S.: L'Apparition de l'infirmité motrice cerebrale et les divers aspects de ce problème. Rev. Neuropsychiat. infant. 16 (1968) 797

Saint-Anne Dargassies, S.: Neurodevelopmental symptoms during the first year of life. Part I.: Essential landmarks for keyage. Part II.: Practical examples and the application of this assessment method to the abnormal infant. Develop. Med. Child Neurol. 14 (1972) 235–264

Saint-Anne Dargassies, S.: Neurological comparison of the two concepts, maturation and development, in the young child. Rev. Neuropsychiat. infant. 22 (1974a) 227–235, 305–334

Saint-Anne Dargassies, S.: Détection sémiologique des troubles du développement neurologique chez le nourrisson jusqu'à 1 an. Rev. Neuropsychiat. infant. 22 (1974b) 305

Saint-Anne Dargassies, S.: Confrontation neurologique des deux concepts: Maturation et développement, chez le jeune enfant. Rev. Neuropsychiat. infant. 22 (1974c) 227

Saint-Anne Dargassies, S.: Neurological Development in Full-term and Premature Neonate. Excerpta Medica, Amsterdam 1977

Schaltenbrand, G.: Normale Bewegungs- und Lagereaktionen bei Kindern. Dtsch. Z. Nervenheilk. 87 (1925) 23–59

Schaltenbrand, G.: Über die Entwicklung des menschlichen Aufstehens und dessen Störungen bei Nervenkrankheiten. Dtsch. Z. Nervenheilk. 89 (1926) 82

Schaltenbrand, G.: The development of human motility and motor disturbances. Atch. Neurol. Psychiat. (Chic.) 20 (1928) 720–730

Schilling, F.: Motodiagnostik des Kindesalters. Marhold, Halle 1970

Schlack, A. G.: Erfassung cerebraler Bewegungsstörungen im 1. Lebensmonat. Dtsch. med. Wschr. 95 (1970) 30

Schröter, W.: Die klinische Behandlung von gefährdeten Neugeborenen. Materia med. Nordmark 67 (1967) 357–363

Schwartz, P.: Alte und neue Beobachtungen über perinatale Schädigungen Neugeborener. Mschr. Kinderheilk. 121 (1973) 264–269

Sellick, K. J., R. Over: Effects of vestibular stimulation on motor development of cerebral-palsied children. Develop. Med. Child Neurol. 22 (1980) 476–481

Semans, S.: The Bobath concept in treatment of neurological disorders. Amer. J. phys. Med. 46 (1967) 732

Sheridan, M.: Infants at risk of handicapping conditions. Mth. Bull. Minist. Hlth. Lab. Serv. Nr. 212 (1962) 38

Sherrington, Ch. S.: Reflex Inhibition as a Factor In the Co-Ordination of Clinical Study to the Physiology of the Cerebral Cortex. Livingstone, Edinburgh 1946

Sherrington, Ch. S.: The Integrative Action of the Nervous System. Cambridge University Press, London 1947

Simons, A.: Kopfhaltung und Muskeltonus. Klinische Beobachtungen. Dtsch. Z. Neurol. Psychiat. 80 (1920)

Soeken, G.: Pathogenese und Differentialdiagnose der cerebralen Bewegungsstörung. In: Diagnose und Therapie cerebraler Bewegungsstörungen im Kindesalter. Bartmann, Frechen 1969

Solomons, G., R. H. Holden, E. Denhoff: The changing picture of cerebral dysfunction in early childhood. I. Pediat. 63 (1963) 113–120

Steinberg, M., J. Rendle-Short: Vestibular dysfunction in young children with minor neurological impairment. Develop. Med. Child Neurol. 19 (1977) 639–651

Stirnimann, F.: Über den Moroschen Umklammerungsreflex beim Neugeborenen. Ann. paediat. (Basel) 160 (1943)

Stutte, H.: Kinder- und Jugendpsychiatrie. In: Psychiatrie der Gegenwart, Bd. II. Springer, Berlin (1960) 955–1076

Tobler, R., E. Köng, I. Hunkeler, K. Preuss: Frühgeborene und cerebrale Bewegungsstörung. Pädiat. Fortbild. Prax. 40 (1974) 44–57

Touwen, B. C. L.: A study on the development of some motor phenomena in infancy. Develop. Med. Child Neurol. 13 (1971) 435–446

Touwen, B. C. L.: The neurological development of the human infant. In: Scientific Foundations of Pediatrics, hrsg. von J. A. Davis, J. Dobbing. Heinemann, London (1973) (S. 615–625)

Touwen, B. C. L.: Neurologische Untersuchung im Säuglingsalter. Pädiat. Fortbild. Prax. 40 (1974) 58–63

Touwen, B. C. L.: Neurological Development in Infancy. Grasmeijer & Wijngaard, Groningen 1975

Touwen, B. C. L.: Early detection of developmental neurological disorders. In: Growth and Development of the Fullterm and Premature Infant. The Jonxis Lectures. Excerpta Medica, Amsterdam 1978

Touwen, B. C. L., H. F. R. Prechtl: The Neurological Examination of the child with Minor Nervous Dysfunction. Clinical Developmental Medicine, 38. Heinemann-Lippincott, London – Philadelphia 1970

Twitchell, T. E.: Normal motor development. J. Amer. phys. Ther. Ass. 45 (1945) 419

Twitchell, T. E.: The neurological examination in infantile cerebral palsy. Develop. Med. Child Neurol. 5 (1963) 271–278

Twitchell, T. E.: Reflex mechanisms and the development of prehension. In: (ed.): Mechanisms of Motor Skill Development, hrsg. von K. Connolly. Academic Press, London 1970 (S. 25–38)

Van Hof, M. W.: Development and recovery from brain damage. In: Connolly, K. J., H. F. P. Prechtl: Maturation and development. Clincs in Developmental Medicine No. 77/78, London: William Heinemann Medical Books, Philadelphia: J. B. Lippincott Co., 1981

Vassella, F.: Die neurologische Untersuchung des Säuglings und Kleinkindes. Pädiat. Fortbild. Prax. 24 (1968) 1–22

Vassella, F., B. Karlsson: Asymmetric tonic neck reflex. Develop. Med. Child Neurol. 4 (1962) 363

Vlach, V.: Ein Screeningtest zur Früherkennung von Entwicklungsstörungen beim Säugling. Pädiat. Prax. 11 (1972) 385–392

Walker, R. G.: An Assessment of the Current Status of the „At Risk" Register. Scot. Hlth. Serv. Stud., Nr. 4, Edinburgh 1967

Walshe, F. M. R.: On disorders of movement resulting from loss of postural tone, with special reference to cerebellar ataxia. Brain 44 (1921) 539

Walshe, F. M. R.: On certain tonic or postural reflexes in hemiplegia with special references to so-called associated movements. Brain 46 (1923) 2–33

Weiss, St.: Studies in equilibrium reaction. J. nerv. ment. Dis. 88 (1938) 160–162

Wiesel, T. N., D. H. Hubel: Single-cell responses in striate cortex of kittens deprived of vision in one eye. J. Neurophysiol. 26 (1963) 1003–1017

Wright, T., J. Nicholson: Physiotherapy for the spastic child: An evaluation. Develop. Med. Child Neurol. 15 (1973) 146

Zappella, M.: The placing reaction in the first year of life. Develop. Med. Child Neurol. 8 (1966) 393–401

Zdańska-Brincken, M., N. Wolański: A graphic method for the evaluation of motor development in infants. Develop. Med. Child Neurol. 11 (1969) 228–241

v. Zglinicki, F.: Die Wiege. Pustet, Regensburg 1979

Zimmer K.: Das Einsame Kind. Kösel, München 1979

Index